"The very fine line between liability and profitability is where drug safety lies on"

Dr. Vera Madzarevic

THE BUSINESS OF CLINICAL TRIALS

Book 1

A compilation of views

By Dr. Vera Madzarevic

2019

Table of Contents

Introduction 11

Clinical Research as a Career. How do You get that very First Job? 15

How do you get the first job in clinical research? 19

Volunteering, entry level jobs and internships in clinical research 27

Catch 22-You Need Experience for Entry Level Clinical Research Jobs 31

Why Women are leading in Clinical Research and Health Care Jobs Globally? 37

What everybody should know about prescription drug safety 39

5 Mistakes to Avoid as a Clinical Trials Monitor 43

Secrets for the Highly Effective Clinical Research Project Manager 49

Four Big Mistakes in Clinical Trials Adverse Event Reporting 53

Who is really monitoring the clinical trial? 59

Should You Quit Your Family for Your Career? 65

7 Reasons Why ePRO Is Not the Solution in Clinical Research (yet) 69

What Everybody Should Know Before Going to a Job Interview 77

Getting Inspired to Make Your Job and Life Better 83

Clinical Research Training Accessibility 87

Do Not Get Caught with Your Pants Down in a Job Interview 91

The Ancient Clinical Research Process 95

The One Mistake in Perception of Drug Efficacy vs. Efficiency 99

The Placebo Effect May Invalidate Our Assumptions 105

7 Reasons Why More Than 85% of Investigational Drugs Fail 111

Clinical Research in a Globally Diverse Population 117

Biotrial Phase I study and the death of a healthy volunteer 121

Where are the clinical research jobs? 125

In Davos (2016) it was said that 5 million jobs will be lost by 2020, will it include clinical research? 133

Should clinical research in academia comply with a different set of standards to be viable? 137

Is your Nursing Job Burning You Out? Have you Though about Clinical Research? 141

Patient Centered Medicine vs. Patient Centric Medicine and vs. Personalized Medicine 145

Depression treatment tools emerging as patient centric medicine is implemented 149

About Pregnancy and Clinical Trials, Really? 151

5 Common Misconceptions for the cause of the Health Care Crisis 159

Opioid overdose due to dose dumping.... 165

Good Clinical Practices (GCP/ICH) R2 Integrated Addendum has changed the Clinical Trials landscape, have you noticed?...167

5 big mistakes in Consenting Clinical Trial Subjects have to do with Vulnerability...169

The New Frontier in Health Care - Artificial Intelligence, a brief opinion 175

Clinical Trials Success Marred with 90% of Disappointment 181

Bringing the hospital care home, a feasible solution for tackling health care costs and promote better outcomes.....185

Quality Management and Risk in Clinical Trials - New GCP R2 Revision...189

Registry Studies and RWD taking the lead in Clinical Research 193

The dawn of The Body of all Knowledge, The natural evolution of Big Data 197

Index 205

Introduction

This book is aimed at clinical research professionals, and other professionals looking into a career in clinical research. Also, people who wants to know about the business of clinical trials can benefit from the reading of this book as it presents a unbiased opinion on matters that affect drug development today.

Clinical research has evolved significantly in the last two decades since the introduction of Good Clinical Practices (ICH-GCP). Regulatory requirements to promote scientifically sound studies while protecting the health and wellbeing of human subjects have been implemented and challenges have risen that questions the process itself and how well people are protected.

However, changes to approaches as is risk-based monitoring and adaptive designs as well as the use of real-world data, have opened the doors to many questions that remain to be answered. The compilation in this book intends to provide an opinion, at least, to the new challenges.

The constant change that clinical research is undergoing, leaves many professionals and public at large wondering about how those will affect the safety of participating subjects and the quality of the data produced.

Clinical research is a multidisciplinary discipline that covers many fields including, pharmacology, ethics, medicine, chemistry, IT, Data management, law, business, and religion among many others.

The XXI century will be marked by deep changes on how we approach life, health and personal choices. Thus, clinical research will be impacted in a manner that we remain to determine yet.

Additionally, it will present challenges based on new optics on gender, equality of opportunities and outcomes. Those changes may affect directly on how clinical trials may be conducted, and how subject rights, safety and wellbeing are going to be protected.

The main reason I wrote this book is to put together my thoughts and opinions regarding specific aspects of clinical research, and many issues regarding professionals who are looking into a career in clinical research. Although most of the topics I already published through my page in LinkedIn, access is limited to its registered users.

In this way, I try to bring to a larger audience different views to common topics, that will allow the reader think further and makeup their own opinions on clinical research and clinical trials.

Enjoy the reading!

Vera M.

14

Clinical Research as a Career. How do You get that very First Job?

When I started my career in clinical research as science professional working for one of the largest pharmaceutical companies and later in contract research organizations, I dedicated myself to gathering and spreading the knowledge on what does it takes to get into a career in Clinical Research. In the late 1980's there were not real programs dedicated to educating clinical research professionals, and information was very limited on what did a career in clinical research entitle. Most people at that time were self-taught, and together with limited industry programs, they gathered the necessary knowledge and experience on the actual job.

As new regulations and international guidelines started taking effect in the 1990's and with standardization on the requirements for submissions to regulatory authorities, research-based companies increased the number of clinical trials and the expenditures on R&D increased accordingly. Together with that growth, a real need for better trained and experienced clinical research professionals developed.

The big question was how to get the right people with the right knowledge and experience to fill all those positions that become available. There was a need for a professional program to fill the gap that would allow professionals with the right background get there.

For that reason, in the early 2000, I developed a very successful program in clinical research that had 23 different courses related to the business of clinical trials. Students from various backgrounds in medicine, science, nursing, and engineering qualified to enter the program. All applicants had the aspiration to become clinical research professionals and did not know where to start. My program allowed them to learn about the profession in record time with real examples and hands on, and quickly were able to get an insight on which jobs they could apply for, build a resume and apply for positions.

What is your background?

Professionals with at least a 4-year degree in medicine, dentistry, biology, biochemistry, pharmacy, nursing and related sciences from recognized institutions are ideal candidates that qualify for a training program in clinical research.

Previous experience in clinical labs, and/or as research scientists/associates enriches the candidate eligibility for a position in clinical research in the future. Any relevant experience can be of advantage to get that very first job.

What a clinical research professional should be?

It is very important to understand that the clinical research professional has to be knowledgeable of local and regional regulations, Good Clinical Practices, the declaration of Helsinki,

Standard Operational Procedures, and basic medical science as is human anatomy, physiology, pathology and pharmacology.

Also, they have to master the abilities to perform their jobs as monitors, auditors or inspectors, data managers, coordinators, investigators, research associates, safety associates and pharmacovigilance, clinical trial supplies associates /supplies managers, etc., and persuade the prospective employer of that.

The clinical research professional must be able to understand all processes involved in clinical research and all the players involved to be part of the conversation.

And the most important, the candidate for a career in clinical research should be:

- eager to learn continuously,
- available to travel extensively,
- able to work long hours,
- able to communicate effectively in person and using the most advanced technologies, and
- be very flexible and adaptable to change in an ever-changing industry, the pharmaceutical clinical research industry.

This article was originally published on March 2, 2015 – edited for this book

How do you get the first job in clinical research?

How do you find that very first job in clinical research?

Getting the very first job in a particular area of your interest is not an easy task, particularly in clinical research (CR). As everything in life, you will need to work very hard for it. There is not magic formula on getting a very first job in clinical research, and there might be different approaches that work for one person, but not for another.

Following, I will give you some tips or key points on how to prepare yourself to be the excellent candidate for that particular job in CR. But, how do you get that very first job in clinical research?

I identified the following key points as critical to prepare for the task of getting that very first job in CR, and I formulated them as questions:

Do you have the background and any related experience?

Do you know what type of job in CR you want to apply for?

> *Are you prepared to get further training and education?*
>
> *Are you ready to tackle the catch-22?*

Answering a question with more questions is not what I intend to do. With the questions above I intend to start a conversation where the points suggested are only a likely path to the objective of landing a job in clinical research.

First, do you have the background and any related experience?

Something you can do very well on your own is to put your experience and achievements in a piece of paper and see if you have what it takes. Your academic and work background are very important to your potential as a clinical research professional. If, for example, you are an ER Nurse looking into the potential of a career change because the long hours and stress do not fit your lifestyle anymore, or you are a basic research scientist who wants to see the other end of your efforts as a researcher, you do qualify for a job in clinical research. However, you need solid training on regulations, GCP, and the clinical research business enterprise. Now, if you background is in art and literature, there is little you can do to qualify for a job in CR unless you have a minor in science that might help you get into a good training program. What about if you are an engineer or an IT specialist? That is another challenge.

Second, do you know what type of job in CR you want to apply for?

To be able to qualify for a job in clinical research, you have to know what people in clinical research do. The following are three of the most common jobs in clinical research that would let you get started.

The Clinical Research Associate or Monitor. The most sought-after job is "The Monitor" of clinical trials. This job is the most common point of entry in clinical research. Nevertheless, it requires experience. So, what does it take to become a clinical research monitor and qualify for a job? Experience. It seems like a catch-22. However, there are many ways of gathering that experience to qualify. I will be discussing about the catch-22 in an upcoming post in a couple of days.

Proper training, and hands on experience are the key to qualify for a CRA job. In the past, large pharmaceutical companies hired science and medical professionals and trained them hands on, in the job, investing great amount of resources to qualify professionals in a career in clinical research. As we approached the 21st century, those jobs started to slide outside of the pharmaceutical industry into a newly created industry of service providers to the pharmaceutical industry, the Contract Research Organizations. Therefore, every new potential employer would like you to work from day one, because the majority of the jobs are in the Contract Research Organizations. These companies are not there to educate or train you in what the job entitles, they want you to do the job for the hours billed to the client. Also, the modality of employment has changed. A long time ago, a CRA used to be a full-time permanent employee of a pharmaceutical company, now that CRA has become a variable in the clinical research budget, where only hours are budgeted. The new CRA is mostly "temporary" or project oriented, they are mostly hourly based than salaried, and the turnaround is very large. That new modality is mostly due to the new business models service companies developed to be cost effective. Nevertheless, there are still few CRA jobs in big pharmaceutical companies, however they are "the few". Your large job market are CROs, and the job requires travel, and many times relocation.

Therefore, a candidate for a CRA job has to be properly trained and educated, with the appropriate background, has to be experienced, willing to travel (sometimes all the time), and be very adaptable to changes in the job market (e.g., take small projects without expecting permanency in a particular appointment).

The Clinical Research Scientist. The clinical research scientist is mostly office based and offers scientific support to the operational aspect of clinical research. This job requires several years of experience in clinical research, where the potential candidate has been involved in clinical trials, and is knowledgeable of the regulatory framework, as well as submission processes, assessments of adverse events and more. Every company may have a different job description for this position, however the common denominator is previous experience in the clinical research business enterprise. Travel is occasional.

The Clinical Research Coordinator. The coordinator is a person responsible for the administration and organizational aspects of a clinical trial at an investigators site. The employer, therefore, is the principal investigator/ hospital/institution where the clinical trial takes place. As such, this job requires a solid background in a related science, medicine, or nursing. Although you do not need to be a registered nurse to do this job, some studies will require from the coordinator to perform certain activities that may require specific training and licenses (phlebotomy, ECG or EEG technician, etc.). Coordinators are also required to know about regulatory requirements, GCP, submissions to ethics committees, and interaction with the sponsor and regulators (FDA, EMA, etc.). Training is very important to become familiar with all the aspects of the job. These jobs are the ideal start point for a nursing professional who is looking for a career change, or for a science professional who cannot compromise on travel as a CRA. The coordinator is not expected to travel, unless is training for a particular study or professional

Third, are you prepared to get training and education?

From my experience, most of the programs in clinical research out there are very theoretical and offer little hands on activities. They are all very expensive too. Academic institutions that deliver programs that provide for MSc. or higher degrees are very robust in information. It is important to highlight that the majority of the programs contribute mainly to the theoretical or academic knowledge of regulations, GCP and ethical aspects of clinical research. Some of them focus on clinical trial design and statistics or make more emphasis on pharmacovigilance or other aspects. The question is, which program you should consider on applying that will give you the ideal balance between the necessary knowledge and experience? The answer is complex, since it depends on what do you want to achieve and how you will use the knowledge acquired.

As I presented in my first post, our company developed a one-year, full time, hands on program that hundreds of medical and science professionals completed in the last ten years. Most of them were very happy with the knowledge and approach to training. Many got their first job when they completed the program, others within months of completing the program, for others it took longer. I had cases where they got jobs even before competing the last part of the program. However, some graduates are still looking. I believe that the same could be said for many programs in clinical research that have the intention to prepare you for the task of getting that first job.

Here is my advice in what you should look for in a program that trains you in clinical research:

1. A proper educational program should last at least 6 months full time or more.
2. A robust program should include practical aspects as is monitoring, auditing, data management, safety reporting, regulatory submissions, and ethics review board approvals, protocol, consent forms and investigational brochures writing, clinical trial budgeting, electronic systems in clinical research, etc. The practical aspect will give you the cutting edge for a job interview.
3. Experience of the instructors. You should be able to know if the instructors are really industry experts or just academics.
4. Hands on training. Find if there are workshops and actual practical application of knowledge, especially for monitoring, auditing, budgeting, safety reporting, etc.
5. Ideally, the program should provide for an internship or hands on exercises/work.

Last, but not least, are you ready to tackle the catch-22?

The catch-22 for the potential candidate for a clinical research job is that the majority of monitoring or coordinating entry level positions require experience. Yes, experience for the entry level position. The minimum experience oscillates between 1 to 3 years. Then, how do you gather experience if to be exposed to a job in clinical research requires minimum experience in that very same job????

Well, that is the catch-22 that I am talking about and that is frustrating so many very qualified candidates. Many qualified professionals cannot get the very first job in Clinical Research because they lack experience in clinical research.

This article was originally published on March 3, 2015 - edited for this book

Volunteering, entry level jobs and internships in clinical research

As part four of my series about clinical research jobs, I dedicate this post to comment about the advantages and disadvantages of volunteering in clinical research in order to gain experience, how it differentiates from an internship and an entry level job.

Before getting engaged into the discussion, I must make it clear that as a volunteer in a clinical research job you want to work to gain experience. It is different from being a volunteer in a clinical trial, since this involves you as the subject of investigation. Please make sure you understand the difference before you start calling sites to work as a volunteer in clinical research. Beware, being a clinical research participant does not give you experience in clinical research that can be translated into a job.

It is very common to believe that volunteering will enhance your resume to make you a more qualified candidate for a clinical research job. Although depends on where in the world you are, volunteering may not be a viable option if you have to support yourself and pay for your college loans. Also, not all institutions will entertain volunteers since they have their own internal policies regarding insurance and employee safety by which they are restricted to allowing non-employees perform any job in the facility.

What volunteering in Clinical Research would help you achieve?

First, some exposure to the clinical research enterprise. Although large pharmaceutical companies and CROs do not entertain volunteers, hospitals may do. So, the fact is that you might volunteer in a health care facility where clinical trials are being conducted. That is a risky approach since all personnel involved in clinical trials has to be qualified by background and experience in clinical trials and that qualification must be properly documented in the clinical trial master files. So again, the story of experience, like the cart before the horse.

Volunteering may represent a good opportunity to learn and get exposure to the job, and to potential employers, but remember that you must state in your resume that you volunteered in a position that gave you the experience in clinical research.

But what would you learn about clinical research in a health care facility as a volunteer?

Unless you have some previous health care experience, you will learn how the health care system works in your area, which are the doctors who are engaged in clinical research and how often they are monitored.

You might also become familiar with the functions of the institutional review board, and their members.

You may have some function in within the clinical research site assisting the coordinator.

Basically, you will start learning about the clinical research enterprise. That also might be translated into a job. But do not keep your hopes to high, generally if a clinical trial site takes in volunteers, is because they do not have the budget to hire someone.

Where do you find volunteer positions?

The majority of teaching hospitals in their web sites have doctors' directories and they may contain a small bio of the doctor where his/her involvement in clinical research is included.

Also, hospitals do take volunteers to assist with the patients. Those volunteer positions are limited and may not be for a clinical research job per se. The best way to get engaged in volunteering is contacting the facilities directly.

Volunteering vs. Internship

In my opinion, an internship is a better option than volunteering since it will focus on you working/learning. You may not generally be paid, and it may cost you time and effort, however it will give you precious experience hands on.

Regardless what you do related to clinical research, you worked on it. Internships may vary from a few weeks to months.

However, do not stay as an intern for more than a year. Move on.

Volunteering vs. entry level job

Of course, you would not be volunteering if you were able to get an entry level job. Yet, I included this section to explain that not all experience has the same value.

If all your clinical research experience is based on a volunteer position you held for few months, make sure that you understood what you were doing as well as put it into perspective when applying for a clinical research job.

Having volunteered to gain experience in clinical research speaks volumes about your willingness to learn and the choice you made for a career in clinical research.

Originally published on March 5, 2015 -edited for this book

Catch 22-You Need Experience for Entry Level Clinical Research Jobs

How do you gain experience if you cannot get the entry level job without it - catch 22?

Experience has been the largest conundrum of highly qualified professionals who want to start a career in clinical research.

The lack of critical day to day hands on experience in the particular tasks the job entitles has closed many doors to prospective candidates oblivious of their own relevant skills.

Here is where I have to bring the concept of what I define as "The Clinical Research Enterprise". Knowledge of the clinical research enterprise is key to get that desired job. Now I am focusing on how to gather experience to get that first job.

What every novice in this industry has to understand is that clinical research is not only a branch of pharmacology or toxicology as academically presented in books. Clinical research is multifaceted discipline combining elements from business, science, medicine and law.

A clinical research professional is a member of that multifaceted world who has to thoroughly understand the business aspect in function of the legal and regulatory framework as well as the market implications and viability of a potential product candidate. This seems to be very complex for the potential candidate to an advertised entry level job, however it holds the real reason behind the conundrum.

Going back to the experience issue. You, as a potential candidate for a clinical research job, have to analyze how compatible is your previous experience in function of the new job you want to apply for. Remember that you must posses a minimum background in science or medicine to consider yourself qualifiable.

There are many ways to present your experience in function of the job sought after. One is relevant experience, the other is direct experience and the last is comparable experience.

Relevant Experience

Besides of your background that has to be compatible with the job you are looking for, you have to present your experience in relevance to the job description presented in the job description. It is not good to regurgitate the keywords in your resume if you cannot put it into context and relevance to your experience and the job you are applying for.

To be able to determine if your experience is relevant to the clinical research job, you must see if the activities/ tasks enumerated in the job description concur with the tasks you preformed in your present or previous jobs.

For example, if you are a critical care nurse and you are willing to get a job as a monitor, you may not have done the actual monitoring of clinical trials for a sponsor, however you have a countless of relevant tasks performed that can translate into an excellent monitor candidate. For instance, you are trained to read patient files and detect safety concerns as well as clinical lab reports in function of determining possible outcomes. You also have experience in navigating the health care system, you are knowledgeable of the disease areas and current marketed drugs. You also may have been exposed directly or indirectly to clinical trials in which your patients were also participating in clinical research and you detected issues regarding the investigated disease or inter-current illnesses. You also are able to proactively interact with medical professionals (as principal investigators) and effectively handle any possible issue regarding patients since that is the daily interaction you have in your job. You have the hands-on experience in completing patient files (electronic or paper based) and understand the information beyond words. You know the challenges principal investigators face in a daily basis, allowing you take steps to avoid oversights in a clinical trial.

As you see, relevant experience may translate into an ideal candidate for a clinical research job, nevertheless, you have to further enhance your knowledge of regulations, GCP, SOPs and the clinical trial process.

Now, if you are a science graduate who wants to work in clinical research, it is advisable that you get the regulatory, GCP and clinical trial process training to be able to interact with the potential employer in an effective manner. Also, you have to gather relevant experience, as for instance your past as a research associate or through graduate training in a relevant area. This relevance is a little weaker, nonetheless depends on how you present yourself and your experience during a job interview.

If you were to have experience as a lab manager, that can translate into knowledge of Standard Operational Procedures, sample handling and storage, temperature controls, good documentation practices, patient privacy, reporting and detecting inconsistencies as well as generating queries to solve inconsistencies. You may have the insight on quality assurance and inspections that may be what the potential employer is looking for.

Direct Experience

Direct experience means that you have done the job and tasks previously for a period of time and can support your eligibility towards that new position. You may have worked as a junior CRA and now you are looking for a more senior position with more responsibilities. You still must demonstrate that you are up to the job and that your experience and background qualifies you.

Comparable Experience

Comparable experience differentiates from relevant experience because you may not have been involved in health care or science recently, but you have a solid academic background and your work experience exposed you to similar processes and procedures. This is a weaker case for experience, but if you are knowledgeable of what the job entitles, you can present your case in a very convincing manner.

Let assume you are a graduate in science with a major in psychology and a minor in biochemistry. However, those paths in life took you to another business direction in which you worked for instance for a law firm and were responsible for writing, editing, filing and archiving documents as well as assisting your superiors in collecting evidence and data regarding cases, and detect inconsistencies.

Your experience makes you a good candidate for either a medical writer or a GCP inspector, from the point of view that you have comparable experience. Now, do not go and apply for jobs yet. You have to enhance your background with training in clinical research in an area that you can excel due to your comparable experience. You have the task to learn about clinical research, rules and regulations, GCP, and the clinical trial process. Once you are aware of the clinical research enterprise, you have to see yourself into which aspect of clinical research you can be suited best and work towards that.

In conclusion, there are three kinds of work experience that might be suitable for the job you are applying for:

DIRECT EXPERIENCE, where you have done previously the job. This experience the majority of entry level candidates do not have.

RELEVANT EXPERIENCE, where you have done similar tasks in the same environment (hospitals, clinics, labs, etc.) and that may suffice for certain potential employers and/or positions if you are able to present it in function of the tasks they require you to perform in clinical research and in the context of the regulatory framework of the clinical research business enterprise.

COMPARABLE EXPERIENCE, where you have gained acuity for very specific tasks that can be easily translated into clinical research, and with further clinical research training may assist you make the case as a candidate for a particular clinical research job.

I believe that this simple post allowed you to see far beyond the catch 22 and tackle the challenge in a positive and constructive manner. Remember, the better trained and familiar with the job you are applying for, the easier will be for you to present your case as of "why should we hire you?", and "what makes you stand-out?"

Originally published on March 4, 2015

Why Women are leading in Clinical Research and Health Care Jobs Globally?

Women are naturally nurturing and compassionate beings, and their selfless dedication to the care of others as well as to medical research are the silver lining of their contribution to the betterment of humanity.

Women are essentially very intuitive and due to better sensibility and compassion, they are able to understand patients...

The majority of clinical research positions, as well as nursing jobs, are filled by women. Women doctors are more common than ever. These careers imply long hours, stress, working under pressure and sacrifice. All these are women qualities and therefore are naturally mostly appealing to them. Women are essentially very intuitive and due to better sensibility and compassion, they are able to understand patients and people at large and perform their jobs more naturally.

Quality over gender has become a determining factor...(for employment)

There are hundreds of articles praising women as CEO's and managers of large companies as well as presidents of countries. Women are also leading in the number of college graduates. These are evidence of the natural progression of women in a society where quality over gender has become a determining factor.

However, we must not forget that women historically are the head managers of the household, one of the most important institutions, making for the economy and well being of their family. At home, women are the wife, the mother, the doctor, the nurse, the cook, the cleaner, the teacher, the lover, the scientist, the policewoman, the clerk, the engineer, the painter, the driver, the plumber, the breadwinner, the daughter, the sister, the everything necessary to make life better.

Women qualities are beyond nationality, religion, race and color.

Women are unarguable suited for leading since leadership is in their nature. Women qualities are beyond nationality, religion, race and color.

Originally published on March 8, 2015 – edited for this book

What everybody should know about prescription drug safety

Introducing to the issue of drug safety

DRUG SAFETY refers to a perception of risk and benefit in function of many variables that depend on the nature of the disease and the outcome expected, as well as on potential liabilities".

These posts about drug safety are written to bring awareness about the issue, and to start a healthy conversation on the topic, bringing also the patients on board to assist the drug development industry and regulators to fine tune on drug related adverse events.

It is needless to say that the pharmaceutical industry has played a major role assisting in the control of diseases that have crippled humanity since the beginning of time. Antibiotics and vaccines are at the forefront of the struggle humanity has to achieve optimal health and reduce suffering.

However, it is interesting to point out that people take for granted that prescription drugs are safe, as long as they use them as indicated by the doctor.

Main issues about drug safety is "perception"

Let's tackle first two important issues:

The first issue here is that the perception of safety has to do with the assumption that if a drug is approved by the FDA, is deemed safe.

It is important to understand that "when the FDA or another health authority deems a drug safe for use in humans, it means that randomized controlled clinical trials (RCT) have been conducted on a selected sample of the patient population for the intended disease, and that it has been demonstrated that, under limited ideal conditions of treatment, the drug had a favorable risk/ benefit ratio." Therefore, patients have to recognize that when they use any medication, prescription or OTC there is an implied RISK. That risk can be foreseeable (because it was observed previously) or unknown (the most important variable in this equation).

Another issue is that people accepts the safety of drugs as per its definition of "free from harm".

The other issue is the implied definition of the word safe, which means free from harm. In the world of pharmaceutical products, a safe product means only that was deemed appropriate for human use, but risks exist, and harm can happen due to the risk involved. Clearly, nothing is 100% safe, even water in large amounts can be toxic. However, prescription or OTC drugs have a more clear potential of risk that we are willing to realize, and proper disclosure to the patient should be provided to make an informed decision on the use of medication.

These assumptions cannot be farther from the reality.

I recently published a book on the matter to answer some of the most common questions people have regarding their prescription drugs. In this part 1, I highlight several key areas about the safe use of prescription drugs:

PATIENT EDUCATION

There is not enough information available in lay language to provide patients with the critical information about the safety of the medications they consume. Conversely, unreliable information circulates in the internet about drug safety. Presently, there are minimal efforts on educating patients about how to correctly assess, take and report about the safety of prescription drugs. The media mostly focus on serious concerns about drugs and vaccines after the fact, where compelling cases speak for themselves. What we hear time and time again is that patients are not aware of all the risks. The truth of the matter is, sometimes we neither. The sample sizes in clinical trials allows us to see only a tip of the iceberg, and the real truth may be somewhat different. Nevertheless, if patients are empowered though education, the risk can be greatly reduced.

PATIENT UNIQUENESS

We all respond differently to drugs, and that depends on intrinsic and extrinsic factors. Since we vary in our genetic makeup, we may react different to drugs, and in the case when a drug has a very limited therapeutic index, risk increases.

THE REALITY

Of the 123.8 million visits to the ER per year in the US, 38% are linked to drug reactions. This means about 47 million ER visits are drug related at a cost of $173 billion US dollars a year.

EFFECTIVE MARKETING

A sense of safety has been attributed to drugs though effective marketing. It is important to understand that the pharmaceutical industry is a business that has to produce drugs (the commodity) that are marketable and profitable. Positioning a drug in the market requires a great effort and large investments, and is time limiting due to the patent lifespan. As such, we, the consumers, have to understand that the marketing approach is to sell a product that is going to satisfy shareholders as well as keeping the company from liability. The very fine line between liability and profitability is where drug safety lies on. Effective marketing is a necessity to keep revenues coming.

> *"The very fine line between liability and profitability is where drug safety lies on"*

As I state in my book 'Are Prescription Drugs Really Safe?', DRUG SAFETY refers to a perception of risk and benefit in function of many variables that depend on the nature of the disease and the outcome expected, as well as on potential liabilities.

Originally published on March 8, 2015 - edited

5 Mistakes to Avoid as a Clinical Trials Monitor

You must have gone through the daily drill of preparing for the monitoring visit countess times. However, you never prepare for unexpected situations that may greatly impact on your performance and the perception of your skills to handle a very stressful situation. Being responsible of a team of monitors and managers, exposed me to countless of situations that can go very wrong unless you are prepared to face them effectively.

With these examples, I intend to assist positively field based clinical trial monitors. The process of formulating the mistake, the consequences and the possible solutions aims at providing a structured approach for easy reading and comprehension.

This post focuses on 5 serious mistakes that every monitor should avoid being able to remain compliant and in good terms with all parties. These are based on years of experience in the matter dealing with issues, sometimes, in uncharted territory.

Mistake #1 – While on monitoring visit, spending your time on the phone dealing with other site issues.

You are very much aware that your visit has been planned very much ahead of time and budgeted by the sponsor and is expected that you dedicate your time at the site working on your site visit. If you are providing services for a CRO, you may be involved on studies for many different sponsors, and dedicating time assigned for one on behalf of solving issues for another will only impact on your performance, where oversights may happen.

That may result on:

- your inability to complete the job in the assigned visit,
- need to reschedule an extra unplanned visit,
- cost overruns
- possible oversight of serious issues due to the lack of time, and
- potential non-compliance

The solution:

- check the call display to verify the caller,
- return the call in an assigned time (e.g. breaks assigned purposely to admin jobs during visits) and,
- make sure that you read all the messages (text and voice) before you respond to a particular call. You may be surprised how many times the coordinator who placed the original call may call again to tell you to "never mind".

Mistake #2 – Write serious observations in the monitoring report without previously discussing the matter or pre-empting your intentions to the principal investigator

It is not uncommon that you may perceive something as a serious issue at a clinical trial site. That may be sometimes your own perception, and with more communication with the coordinator and involving the investigator, you will have a better insight on the concern. For example, source documents are not available for you to verify. Those documents may be filed elsewhere due to the document management system at the facility, however they were not provided to you at the visit. Guiding the site personnel on what do you need instead of just flagging it and reporting it as non-compliance to the sponsor, will allow to clear the matter in a moment time without hard feelings.

That may result on:

This mistake can cost you the much-needed good relationship with the site personnel. However, if the issue reoccurs, you may have to change your strategy and recommend more training to the site personnel.

The solution:

- Always try to solve issues amicably.
- Open ways of communications with the site.
- Make sure that the site is aware of your observations

Mistake #3 – Take things in your own hands

It is sometimes very frustrating to see that a site makes the same mistakes again and again and that you are pointing out the same things every visit. So, to avoid again the same talk with your coordinator or investigator, you do the job for them. This is a very dangerous precedent, since the coordinator will expect in the future that you keep doing it. Your job should be pointing out at concerns, verifying data and that patients are safe, making sure that the site adheres to the protocol and compiles to regulatory requirements. Your job is not to do things for the site to avoid non-compliance issues. It wastes your time and puts a lot of stress on you. If the site does not have enough personnel to do the job, make sure to stress that in the monitoring report as well as the delays that lack of resources is producing.

That may result on:

- Burn out
- Cost overruns
- Oversights
- Reduced performance

The solution:

- Make sure that the site has been properly trained
- Make sure that the investigator has real time available to do the expected job
- Suggest methods to save time and be more effective
- Be of assistance, but do not take things in your own hands.

Mistake #4 – Confronting your Principal Investigator/coordinator with suspicion of fraud or misconduct

Eventually, you may be faced with challenges like this one in your career and is not an easy one. If you suspect fraud or misconduct at a site, NEVER confront the site personnel or the principal investigator. First, make sure that you are aware of your company procedures on how to deal with fraud and misconduct. Also, collect as much evidence you can (photocopy documents, gather opinions form site personnel regarding issues or inconsistencies, ask site personnel for their own concerns), and document everything. Fraud and misconduct are very serious and should never be handled unprepared.

That may result on:

- Serious confrontations
- Unfounded accusations based on your perception
- The investigator assuming a defensive position

The solution:

- Your suspicion of fraud or misconduct may not always be founded, it may happen that the site is just sloppy and disorganized. Focus on collecting information.
- Follow your company procedures for that matters, and inform your superiors
- Keep cool, and do not engage in discussions at the site

Mistake #5 – Sharing work space with another monitor from another company

Although a no brainier, it does happen. It is understandable that you are willing to accommodate your investigators time and space, however sharing space with another monitor is not something you should compromise for.

Make sure that your site understands that you are dealing with confidential information and that you are not supposed to handle confidential material (source documents, protocols, patient's lists or data) in the presence of not authorized personnel.

The same applies when you are not there, you expect that the site keeps all the documentation pertaining your study confidential.

This mistake may result on:

- Disclosure of patients personal and confidential information to unauthorized persons
- Access to confidential industrial information to the competition

- Inability of doing your job because of the above
- Reduced performance
- Non-compliance

The solution:

- Announce your visit in advance and clearly state your requirements from day 1
- If you are confronted with the challenge on the spot, if space cannot be provided, reschedule your visit
- Provide for training to your site regarding confidentiality of clinical trial records
- All these mistakes are not uncommon and are the source of many issues regarding your ability to conduct effective site visits.

Originally published on March 9, 2015

Secrets for the Highly Effective Clinical Research Project Manager

It feels good when you can share your experience and knowledge to help other professionals in the same arena improve their own skills. Much more is the anticipation when that improvement can be easily translated to success and savings for your company (win/win).

First, let me define what a Highly Effective Project Manager is. He/she is the person responsible of the entire oversight of the clinical trial project and its proper implementation on time and within the budget (taking into account that the timeliness and the budget were properly established in the first place). To be considered a highly effective clinical research project manager, your experience in the clinical research enterprise has to be vast and real. I consider that anything less than 5 years of hands on monitoring experience at different levels, would not allow you to gasp all the variables in function of the real potential issues that may arise and hinder the success of your company project.

The Highly Effective Project Manager builds effectiveness around time and money in function of the desired outcome

Remember, the keywords on this conversation are "on time" and "within budget".

I highlighted two key issues that are the main factors in project failures (time and money). The highly effective project manager builds effectiveness around them.

Secret #1: **BECAME AWARE** - Reduce the unknowns to the minimum during the planning process and include the higher risk due to new unknowns as a variable in the calculation of timelines and budget. As a Clinical Research Project Manager, you should be extremely cautious in the planning process, especially if you are assigned to run clinical trials in new indications or with very innovative products where not only you, but nobody has experience.

Secret #2: **BE REAL** - Making/breaking point analysis with estimation of most realistic plan

Do not try to impress your director/superiors by underestimating budgets and planning very tight timelines and limited resources. As well as, do not overestimate timelines, budget and resources just "to be in the safe side".

Unfortunately, in clinical research, some rules are different than in any other industry. Mainly, there is a limit on how much money and resources you can put in a project with the aim at reducing time to completion and increase the probability of success. (The limiting factor is that we are depending on human physiology and pathology to measure response, and that will follow the rules of nature). Therefore, we have what I call a the "breaking point" in project planning in which regardless of resources and money, we reach a plateau in the outcome.

Also, I established something I call a "making point" in project planning in which there is a minimum of budget resources and estimated time to completion that you could achieve. We can calculate the making point utilizing the critical path analysis, we can review the calculations to optimize them further. That is an ideal plan (with cost, resources, and timelines) that seldom exist in the real world, however it is good to have the idea for analysis and planning purposes.

A wise decision between the making and the breaking points (that include critical variables as is cost, timelines and resources, as well as include all the unknowns and the higher risks) should be made by the highly effective manager to bring the project to success. In this case, that decision will not be the result of application of another project management tools, as for instance is PERT and consider yourself happy. But to rationalize as well as incorporate many more variables and factors from real experience (not assumptions) provided by more observers and collaborators in the planning (see the secret #3)

Secret #3: **LISTEN and LEARN**- Discuss your project plan with the team and other managers, and include feedback before running into problems

Present your project plan to your team and other project managers that may be more experienced and include everyone that has a critical task assigned to provide their feedback on the feasibility of the project. The latter are the ones implementing your project plan, and they may have a different approach to the tasks and timelines. A highly effective project manager listens to their team and peers, and values their contribution.

Of course, I have hundreds of tips and recommendations, and I can go on all day. However, I consider these three secrets key in the planning phase of a project. With accurate planning, and proper ongoing re-evaluation, there is no need to incur in cost overruns and jeopardize and entire study or the development of a new drug.

Originally published on March 10, 2015

Four Big Mistakes in Clinical Trials Adverse Event Reporting

Every monitor of clinical trials faces the challenges to determine whether all adverse events were reported to the sponsor. Clinical Trials have two main endpoints, one is efficacy and the other safety, being both of them of equal importance from the regulatory standpoint. Unreported or underreported adverse events are a major problem during regulatory inspections. The monitor has the responsibility to capture any issue with reporting before the inspector does and ensure compliance.

Adverse event (AE) is an absolute term in function to Good Clinical Practices, defined as "… any untoward medical occurrence in a patient or clinical investigation subject (when) administered a pharmaceutical product and that does not necessarily have a causal relationship with this treatment". This is different from the definition of adverse drug reaction (ADR) that is "…all noxious and unintended responses to a medicinal product related to any dose (…) means that a causal relationship between a medicinal product and an adverse event is at least a reasonable possibility…"

Having clarified the terms, all adverse events in clinical trials should be reported regardless of relationship and investigators (PI) have to be made aware that reporting is mandatory. Many times, we are faced with investigators or sponsors opinions contrary to the requirement mainly because they "assume" and that becomes part of common mistakes in AE reporting.

Note that the analysis of the mistakes below are in function of GCP and do not entertain opinions that may be interpreted otherwise during an inspection.

Mistake #1 "It's not an adverse event, it is a common progression of the disease"

Monitors may become oblivious of an AE in a clinical trial, because they are not even collected when considered by the investigator as a common progression of the disease.

I have heard this opinion hundreds of times, where investigators as well as sponsors "assume" that if it is disease related, it should not be reported. Many ethics committees also sides with that opinion to reduce the burden of reviewing all the reports. However, there is a good rationale for reporting all AE in a clinical trial regardless of the relationship.

First, a clinical trial is an experiment that tries to demonstrate a hypothesis. Is not medical care.

Second, if the clinical trial is blinded, regardless of the treatment groups, there is no possibility that the PI could make the assertion that is not reportable because is the common progression of the disease. What if the study treatment (drug/comparator) is responsible for further accelerating the common progression of the disease? What if that is an early indicator of lack of efficacy? we could never conclude that because the data is not available.

Lastly, the challenge of "filtering "which AE are going to be reported, biases the safety analysis, downplaying the safety of the product, regardless of what originally could have been agreed with the regulator. Many protocols even establish which adverse events are not going to be collected.

Mistake #2 "It's not a new AE, it's the same AE but a bit more severe"

It is obvious that the safety profile of a study drug is going to look weaker if all AE that worsen in time are reported as a new adverse event. The worsening of the severity of an adverse makes it a NEW adverse event. It is very common that monitors overlook this fact, not requiring the PI to report the adverse event that by virtue of severity as a new one instead of the same old one that is ongoing.

Mistake #3 "Lab results are automatically categorized as normal and abnormal by the testing facility, therefore the investigator might not re-classify them further as AEs"

In most of the cases, monitors do not challenge a lab abnormality classification, as well as the investigator only review the lab results in function of the safety of the patient, but not classify abnormalities because considers that all was already electronically classified and submitted by the lab automatically. They might occasionally override an abnormal classification to allow patient eligibility in a clinical trial when the value is not significant.

Here we have several issues

First, that the monitor and the investigator may assume that all lab abnormalities have already been classified by the lab, therefore they do not include the clinically significant ones as AE in the report

Second, that lab abnormalities are not all AE, and further classification as clinically significant and insignificant is to be performed by the PI. Lab abnormalities are mostly an overridden value by the investigator in function of significance to ensure enrollment

Following are the responsibilities in reporting and verification

The investigator is responsible to assign significance to all lab abnormalities and report them in the Case Report Form.

The monitor should review the lab report, and the classification made by the investigator ensuring that lab AEs are properly reported and classified.

If lab AE are overridden by the PI, the monitor should investigate and document further to avoid non-compliance. If the lab abnormality meets exclusion, the monitor should procure patient withdrawal.

Lab results are the bulk of safety data, and proper review, classification and reporting should be ensured to avoid overlooking safety signals.

Mistake #4 – "The adverse event is not related to the study drug"

For an adverse event (AE) relationship to study treatment is not relevant in function of reporting by nature of its definition. Nevertheless, we encounter investigators and also sponsors classifying AE as not related to the study treatment without unbinding in function of pre-established rules in the protocol. That misinterpretation in the definition of AE reporting brings up the issue of how to ensure that all AE are reported.

All AE's should be further classified in function of its relationship to study treatment once the codes are open (in the case of blinded studies) and proper consultation with the investigator and sponsor experts should be sought and documented.

In my opinion, AE drug causality can be assessed either as

- Certain or related, where, event or laboratory test abnormality, with plausible time relationship to drug intake, cannot be explained by disease or other drugs response to withdrawal plausible (pharmacologically, pathologically), event definitive pharmacologically or phenomenologically (i.e. an objective and specific medical disorder or a recognised pharmacological phenomenon), re-challenge satisfactory, if necessary
- Probably/likely, event or laboratory test abnormality, with reasonable time relationship to drug intake, unlikely to be attributed to disease or other drugs, response to withdrawal clinically reasonable, re-challenge not required
- Possibly related, event or laboratory test abnormality, with reasonable time relationship to drug intake, could also be explained by disease or other drugs, information on drug withdrawal may be lacking or unclear
- Unlikely, event or laboratory test abnormality, with a time to drug intake that makes a relationship improbable (but not impossible), disease or other drugs provide plausible explanations.

If we review all the options carefully, the definitions never allow complete disambiguation that the drug in question might have not played a role in the AE. Therefore, we can have different opinions varying from high certainty to low certainty. The causality of AE classification is done in function of the medical opinion of the investigator and in concurrence with the sponsor through the study monitor. Nevertheless, may not be acceptable for the regulator.

The causality of AE classification is done in function of the medical opinion of the investigator and in concurrence with the sponsor through the study monitor. Nevertheless, may not be acceptable for the regulator.

It is very important for the monitor to verify documentation behind the investigators classification before they concur, especially when unlikely is the option. The reason behind it is to allow further reassessment when the clinical trial/study report is written and when submission of safety data is performed.

Also, it is very important to make sure that adverse events do not go unreported or underreported because of an inadequate causality assessment. That may be a red flag in an inspection.

it is very important to make sure that adverse events do not go unreported or underreported because of an inadequate causality assessment. That may be a red flag in an inspection.

Remember that from the legal standpoint, as far as there was study drug in the patient's circulation during the event, a negative causality assessment would impact on the legal opinion that the drug might not have a role in the AE.

From the legal standpoint, as far as there was study drug in the patient's circulation during the event, a negative causality assessment would impact on the legal opinion that the drug might not have a role in the AE.

Originally published on March 12, 2015

Who is really monitoring the clinical trial?

Clinical Trial Monitoring is one of the most important activities in clinical research, involving the collaborative as well as synergistic effort of many parties. Although the clinical trial monitor or CRA, which is assigned by the sponsor has the responsibility to check for compliance and patient safety through mainly on site monitoring visits, we have several layers of monitoring that also have their share of responsibility in detecting noncompliance and safety issues. Sometimes, those are not properly attributed in regulatory inspections, relying most of the responsibilities onto principal investigators.

It is important to bring awareness on who those parties are, how they interact and how the data is verified and scrutinized by them.

The first question is who the parties involved in monitoring clinical trials are. The answer is based on the responsibilities of the main players in clinical research according to Good Clinical Practices, and is as follows:

Medical Monitoring: The Investigator (formally independent from all parties, but financially dependent from the sponsor)

Compliance Monitoring and Data verification : The Monitor/CRA (assigned by the sponsor and dependent of the sponsor company)

Overall and Individual Safety Monitoring: The Independent Data Safety Monitoring Committees (mainly contracted by the sponsor- but independent in functions)

Safety and Ethical monitoring: The Independent Ethics Committees (totally independent form the others)

Medical Monitoring

The clinical trials investigator (principal investigator) is responsible for the medical monitoring of the patients enrolled in the study at the site. As such, the investigator role does not end when the subject is enrolled and met criteria for inclusion (therefore patient based data reporting cannot be a tool that replaces the PI, since it exposes the patients to unknown risks without professional interaction, however it can properly supplement it). The PI role includes continuous assessment of patient health and safety while in the clinical trial. This means that the PI, regardless that are specialist in one particular area of medicine investigating a specific drug, is responsible of the overall health of the subject. That responsibility emanates from the Declaration of Helsinki and is further included in GCP/ICH and tacitly implied in regulations. This means basically, that the PI is the only contact with the patient sponsor has.

Compliance Monitoring and Data verification

The responsibility of the CRA or monitor (assigned by the sponsor) is to determine, among other things, that the source data is available and that the data submitted reflects the source, as well the monitor is responsible to determine that reporting of clinical trials safety information is accurate and that the study is conducted according the protocol. The monitor in this case is the main link between the site and the sponsor and must ensure that the study is fully compliant to regulations. Therefore, site interaction in the form of the physical visit must exist, since this verification also involves the continuous eligibility of the clinical trial site. Once data is verified, the data passes a next layer of scrutiny.

Overall and Individual Safety Monitoring

Independent Safety Monitoring Committees or Data Safety Monitoring Boards were envisioned to provide an extra layer of important safety data monitoring for the overall study and product development. Since monitors are not able to observe the big picture of safety in a study because they are only exposed to a very small fraction of subjects, these committees review all data as submitted in a blinded or un-blinded fashion depending on the strategy selected by the company. Also, we have to understand that since monitoring become an outsourced activity where dedicated monitoring is not possible, outsourced monitors provide services for many sponsors and serve several studies at the same time and therefore not immersed and aware of all subjects involved. This layer of monitoring depends on the quality and reliability of the data submitted from any source (investigator site, patient reported outcomes data, labs, etc.). These committees must be properly setup with clear standard operational procedures and trial rules for safety detection and reporting.

Safety and Ethical Monitoring

Ethics committees (EC) were also granted with the responsibility to monitor the safety of subjects of a study at the site they gave approval or are responsible to. The physical monitoring visit by ethics committee members is unusual. Those committees have the responsibility to review in a timely manner, all safety reports (internal and external) to further determine in a continuous fashion if the study can carry on at the site. The effectiveness of their review depends on the quality of the safety reports as well as the reporting timelines. Also, their expertise and expeditious reviews are important. EC have a great responsibility towards their site (they are the site gate keepers), nevertheless, their members may not be properly trained on the reality of working under specific procedures and regulatory requirements and lack of effective quality assurance to guarantee compliance in operation and implementation of SOPs and regulatory requirements.

In summary

These four levels of oversight should work in concert to be able to guarantee patient safety and data quality.

The investigator is the first level guaranteeing the health and well-being of the subjects enrolled

The ethics boards are the gatekeepers, they have the power of revoking approval if they consider that patent safety is in jeopardy and/or ethically the study cannot either start or continue.

The monitors are the eyes and ears of the sponsor and have the responsibility to validate reported data and study compliance.

The data safety monitoring board, being empowered with all safety and efficacy data of a trial or a drug per se according to the protocol, SOPs and pre-established rules, have the responsibility to analyze that data in a timely manner, flag safety concerns and react informing the sponsor promptly of any concerns that may expose subjects to a higher risk as determined in the protocol.

All of these layers of oversight depend on the first step, and that is the ability of the investigator to capture the right information and submit data promptly for assessment to the other layers. Therefore, the PRINCIPAL INVESTIGATOR is the weakest link in this process, and more efforts have to be invested providing for proper training and education. There is an evident disconnect between the sponsor regulatory might and the investigators responsibilities at the site, where they are left to fend themselves off in case that an inspection comes with observations that prompt obligatory responses.

Originally published on March 15, 2015

Should You Quit Your Family for Your Career?

The balancing act....

I just read a post by Paul Drury where he asks the opposite question of whether you should quit your career for your family, and it touched me very hard. Instead of commenting on his post, I wanted you know of what my experience was, and how I tackle the question, but the other way around. One thing I want to clarify, that a career is not a job that you may hold, but the path in a profession that you choose to walk.

I spent almost 15 years in my post secondary education, achieving every bit of success you could dream of, awards, scholarships, fellowships, becoming a PhD at 25, focusing on my post PhD work overseas and going after my profession. My drive to make a difference in this world took me to almost every center of excellence in Europe and the US. I was at the summit of my career, financially and otherwise independent, I was going places. As I learnt from early age, re-evaluation of my goals as a human being are the most important thing, I have to dedicate my time to.

Drawing a potential path, re-evaluating it continuously was the key to get where I am now. I had to face huge challenges, especially being a woman in a man's world and having to go through pregnancies and storms of body changes and keep my smile.

To keep focused and guarantee my success, I put myself into the path of the pursuit of happiness, not money. In my opinion, financial compensation by itself its only a decoy for happiness. I wanted to grow stronger and wiser giving a meaning for me being here in this world at this time.

Having a family was the natural path of my existence, regardless what is my profession is. Achieving completeness means to fulfill the objective of being. Remember that the measure of success depends on the measuring tool you choose and the metrics you use.

Therefore, I affirm,

YOU SHOULD NOT QUIT YOUR CAREER FOR YOUR FAMILY!!!

but you have to,

REDEFINE YOUR CAREER WITHIN YOUR FAMILY

Flexibility and redefinition of your roles as a professional should be the rule instead of exception.

The markets change continuously, and we have to re-adapt to change, but let's put that into our advantage, and put our family into the equation.

When your children are very small, they need mommy/daddy time. As they grow, they will be needing more time with other kids, and then as soon as you blink, they are all grownup giving you advise on how to live your own life. That is the cycle of life, in which your career as a professional has to find a niche that will achieve a dual objective, your personal happiness and your professional satisfaction.

Remember that the measure of success depends on the measuring tool you choose and the metrics you use.

I will never forget the day I was filing for my maternity benefits, I read a sign that said..."by the year 2000 most of professionals will be self-employed or work for a small business...", and I said to myself, OK I will take the challenge.

It was not easy to leave the corporate world, big salaries, travel, interaction with great minds. However, I used it to my advantage because these big corporations need consultants and they outsource most of their work.

I founded my own company in the year 2000, and with three beautiful kids in tow, I worked around them and their time. I scheduled meetings when they were in school during those core hours, and I used every technology available to run my business. I kept the business size to manageable with my family. I did not grow to a size that would take me to a position where I have to dedicate them less time they were entitled to. While they were at home, mommy does not work, mommy is mommy attending to their needs. While they are asleep or in school, mommy works. I even included them in my business to give them some insights on what work is. Did I have sleepless nights? yes. Did I wonder where would I be had I not taken this path? yes. Do I have any regrets, NO!

They are all grown up now, everyone heading towards their own destinies, I am still working around their needs and time, supporting them in the quest for their own happiness, but now I am harvesting the fruits of my efforts.

Originally published on March 19, 2015

7 Reasons Why ePRO Is Not the Solution in Clinical Research (yet)

The challenge

The use of smartphones is widespread and has a pivotal role in peoples life in the 21st century. Looking around we can see everyone staring at their phones, like there is the solution to all our problems. Smart devices opened a huge window of opportunity for the collection of health information like never before. Clinical trial platforms like electronic patient reported outcomes (ePRO) have already proven a very useful tool in replacing patient diaries. Sometimes companies have gone further and collected critical efficacy and safety data with the ePRO platform. However, this is the first time that a manufacturer of smartphones has found an new niche in medical research providing for an open sourced health data platform.

Many of you have already became aware of Apple® getting into the business of health research providing for a very powerful tool called ResearchKit™. Microsoft® also had an incursion a while ago with data base solutions. Although a great idea and a preview of things to come, we have to become more critical of the new tools that promises too much without consideration of the regulatory environment. This particular tool may be ideal for registry studies as well as some phase IV studies, however it is too early to consider it applicable to phases I-III of clinical research.

In my opinion, electronic tools to collect data directly from the patient has excellent applications in medical practice and at bedside, as well as for the collection of biometrical data in clinical trials that is prone to errors in the process assessment and recording. Basically, I consider that properly validated systems of direct data collection is a blessing for medical and research purposes.

Nevertheless, the clinical research process is very complicated, and ePRO may not be a solution for all aspects in clinical research.

Going back to the ResearchKit by Apple, they say in a press release issued on March 9, 2015…"ResearchKit also makes it easier to recruit participants for large-scale studies, accessing a broad cross-section of the population—not just those within driving distance of an institution. Study participants can complete tasks or submit surveys right from the app, so researchers spend less time on paperwork and more time analyzing data. ResearchKit also enables researchers to present an interactive informed consent process. Users choose which studies to participate in and the data they want to provide in each study" …

Also, these type of applications although open source, rely on Apple iPhone IOs, for now, what makes the market limited to iPhone users. This, by itself, introduces selection bias of subjects in clinical research, depriving the opportunity from participation to less affluent people.

The reasons

Let's look at why we should not utilize ePRO systems as a solution in clinical research without getting into a regulatory, ethical or legal quagmire.

Subject procurement. The process of subject procurement and selection is very critical and procuring subjects with ads in Facebook or other social networking platform opens a can of worms. Why? Very simple, people do not understand the clinical research process, most consider clinical trials as an option to get medical care for free, and many may consider it as a form of income.

Social media is a public platform that does not support patient privacy requirements.

Utilizing people's data (with weak consenting processes) into a Big Data platform to search for potential clinical trial subjects, may bring up ethical and legal issues of great proportions as are privacy, confidentiality, access rights, etc.

People may use the same platform to voice their concerns about the clinical trial or start posting updates on their health status in social media or on their walls as the study progresses, violating confidentiality and blindness.

Subject selection (and screening). Choosing the right subjects is critical to the reliability of the results in a clinical trial. A scenario that is in the make, is to develop a tool with all the right questions to have potential subjects screen themselves as if they were to determine their eligibility to participate in a study. Then that data can be pooled into Big Data with all the information we have about that subject (gathered from social media, and why not, electronic health records accessed with the consent of the subject, something the subject did by pressing the button "accept" and may not be fully aware of the implications) to determine further their eligibility. We also can send them do a blood test to include that as data in the selection process. This scenario, as presented, is marred with red flags. The most important thing is that before any data pertaining the clinical trial is collected (regardless of the form) a proper informed consent has to be read, understood and signed. The consenting process is more that clicking "accept to the terms and conditions" (I will go back to this in the point 7). Let's assume the subject accepted to go through the process of selection, then the subject is the one answering the screening questionnaire, not a qualified health professional. The subject perception on his/her condition, although valid, is not qualified and therefore it cannot be utilized as selection data for further enrollment unless a qualified investigator verifies the information. However, let's assume it was accepted as valid data, that subject was selected as a potential clinical trial participant.

Subject enrollment. It is important to remark that only the qualified investigator is the one who has the responsibility and authority to enroll subjects in a clinical trial because according to his/her qualified opinion, the subject fulfills all the pre-established criteria in the protocol and is fit to participate in a study. However, if we were to rely on ePRO systems for this job, the process of subject enrollment will be done by a computer algorithm that "determined" that the subject meets all the inclusion and none of the exclusion criteria taking into account the screening data provided by the subject themselves and the Big Data framework utilized to analyze that patient eligibility. Although this process will allow screening and enrollment of huge amount of subjects in a very short time and with minimum resources, it is completely contrary to the requirements of the FDA 21CFR312, GCP/ICH, EU REGULATION No 536/2014 and the Declaration of Helsinki.

Subject randomization. These systems consider that collecting health data including lab data, and analyzing it utilizing validated algorithms can provide for very accurate patient selection and further those selected subjects are randomized into blinded treatments where, electronically, a subject is assigned treatment. In practice that will look something like this in the patient's smartphone or tablet: "You've been selected!" your study medication will arrive in the mail soon. Real time instructions will be provided to you once the medication is delivered". It also can have a disclaimer that says "if you have any question, our automated system is available 24/7 to answer, you can also have a live chat with one of our experts" (outsourced, of course). This can be achieved right now with systems implemented for commercial activities. Imagine, having thousands of subjects, and only one "virtual site"... that is "science fiction". Also, here we have flying all the regulatory red flags very high and emergency bells too! Basically, although some aspects may comply with 21CFR11, subjects' safety will be highly compromised and access to care will be very limited, whereas subjects will be referred to ER if they develop a serious adverse event. Wow, we got rid of the principal investigator, the coordinator, the site, the pharmacist and drug accountability, also source documents will not exist or have to be verified because is either patient reported or electronically captured. We will not need monitors because there will not be data to verify nor actual site to visit.

Drug dispensing. The process would be fully automated and prompted by the algorithm in the Big Data system and the clinical trial supply management system will take care of that. It is important to understand that drug dispensing has to be done by a qualified professional and that the subject should be properly instructed on the use of the investigational product, and all that should be properly recorded at the site. Delivering study medication automatically may not comply with any of these requirements.

Investigational product may be delivered to the wrong person, what about the accountability at that point?

Subject visits. With a fully integrated ePRO system, as I am presenting here, the subject will have only virtual visits in the form of periodical interaction with the phone/tablet to answer questions, provide for some biometrics supported by the device, and perform blood tests in a lab. Therefore, the subject does not need to live close to a clinical trial site, they can be anywhere. Again, in clinical trial phases I-III, this approach will not stand the test of the regulation requiring the principal investigator to assess the safety and efficacy of the intervention as well as ongoing eligibility of the subject in the clinical trial, and to have physical visits to the site. I agree that these virtual site visits can be performed for collection of additional data and as an additional resource as a patient diary, however it cannot replace the collection of critical safety and efficacy data by a qualified professional.

Subject consenting. The consenting of a subject is not the signing of a document, but a process by which a subject is informed by a 'qualified professional' of all the relevant information about the investigational product risk, benefit, options, and the trial itself. It is a process were subjects ask questions, goes home and thinks, returns and eventually signs. All the process must be fully documented as per regulatory requirements in the patients file. Pressing a button of "accept" at the end of the electronic consent document may not fulfill the requirement of proper information, discussion, time to evaluate, and agreement.

If that process is replaced by an eConsent in which the subject is provided for all the information and is asked to press "accept" if they agree to the terms and conditions, it is not only non-compliant to regulatory requirements, but undermines the importance of providing education to the subject during the process, as well as support for the proper understanding of the clinical trial. It is important to highlight that very few subjects, once reading the information in the consent, do actually sign.

In summary, I consider that we are very far from an eTrial, in which all data is generated outside of the clinical trial site, non-verifiable, where subjects are seldom faced with an actual doctor who will assess their condition, and provide for qualified medical support during a clinical trial. In order to moving away from the complicated and burdensome clinical trial process, as it stands now, we will need a complete reconsideration of regulations, deep changes in the process of how health care is delivered, ensuring that the established guarantees, rights and protections to subjects prevail in function of a streamlined eProcess.

The solution

I believe that great companies like Apple, as well as an exceptional CEO as Tim Cook, to further guarantee their incursion in health research, should question why the clinical research process is so complicated, and why is not getting better, easier, faster or cheaper. Those questions should be directed to us, clinical research industry professionals, to have the complete picture of what is needed to streamline research without compromising patient safety and data reliability while remaining compliant. Having a better insight about regulatory constraints will allow developers work towards a real solution that will be more palatable for the industry as well as regulators.

I am open to provide critical insights on this exciting new world of eClinical Research, are you?

Originally published on March 28, 2015

What Everybody Should Know Before Going to a Job Interview

I was recently interviewing a potential candidate for a job, when the conversation veered towards how the candidate relates to other employees at work. It is important to mention that I am talking about a young and very successful man, with all the necessary attributes to succeed in life, but something in the perceptions regarding how he relates to others seem not right. He said…"all the other employees in my division are my friends"…"we go to lunch together, sometimes I play tennis with some, we took pictures together and some of them post that picture on.."…and he got me there.

I started evaluating what was incorrect in the assertions I was being showered with, and I found myself like listening my own kids expressing themselves. This person did not know the difference between the people he relates to and the level of trust, confidence and reliance he can expect from them when relating.

What do I mean with that?

Simple, youth nowadays, cannot differentiate a friend, from a colleague, a classmate, a peer and an acquaintance. I came to the conclusion that after that very long interview, the misty level of understanding of what degree of relationship youth have with each other and other people at large, and therefore the level of trust, confidence and reliance is skewed by the Facebook button "friend". To this person, and many people presently, a friend is the person that they accepted on Facebook, and also have indirect conversations with (virtual or real). The only thing expected from a "friend" is to share his/her FB page, or basically nothing relevant, a friend basically become everyone known (factually or virtually) and interact directly or indirectly. By extension, everyone else they know are "friends".

This new concept of "friend" distorts the way relationships are perceived and expectations met, and further may skew the way people approaches each other.

I consider that, having to go through the gruelling process of interviewing loads of candidates, that a thorough clarification of how people relates to each other will allow interviewers understand your qualities, strengths and weaknesses.

Who is who?

Let's start with "Friend"

You highest level of relation to a person that is not a relative is a FRIEND. The level of trust, confidence and reliance should be the highest. Only few people in your life would qualify as a friend, and then things may happen to make them drop from the friendship zone. Then you realize that they were never your friends. The friend is your confident, your buddy, and your shoulder to lean on. You will be lucky if you have just a few friends in your lifetime. That is why, when people talk about that they have thousands of friends (on Facebook), basically they have thousands of people looking at their page (that you allowed or not, if public) and they do not fulfill any of the attributes described above.

In an era of virtual interactions where people are interacting even while sleeping just because somebody contacted their page in social media, is not considered relevant or of quality.

The next level is "Colleague"

You are a colleague with people you share your job with and is about the same pay level, otherwise they are either your boss or your subordinate. You have a lot of things in common with a COLLEAGUE. You may feel prompted to share your personal problems, and your personal life, beware, he/she is a colleague, you did not choose each other and you are compelled due to your job to be together and interact positively. While in your job, you are with this person, and you may not see him/her again when you change jobs or positions. Therefore, your level of expectations from a colleague are accordingly to the job you have to fulfill. Getting too friendly with a colleague may open you to share weaknesses that in turn can be used against you in the rat race.

Can a colleague become a friend? that only time will tell. It may, but there are too many conflicts of interest in the way (e.g. promotions, bonuses, salaries, etc.). You can be friendly with a colleague but not consider him/her a friend.

Then is the "Classmate"

Here is where the majority of the Facebook friends fall on. Youth considers most CLASSMATES as friends, and they are not as such. You share a lot of time with them, you grow with them, they know each other's weaknesses and strengths, but they do not develop any meaningful relationship since the interactions are due to the fact that they share a classroom, they are about the same age, may share the dorm, and study together. Can a classmate become a friend? Probable, but only time will tell.

Following is a "Peer"

A PEER is a person who is equal to your abilities, qualifications, age, background and social status. Peers are not considered as friends, nor colleagues, they are your equals to which you can have meaningful conversations without getting personal or collegiate. Those are people that can judge your abilities and support your knowledge and capabilities.

The last step in the level of relationship is *the "Acquaintance"*

The ACQUAINTANCE is someone you know, as the mailman, or the gardener, even the security person at work. You know that person because you have certain interactions due to your work, school or needs. They are not considered your friends. You can address to them as people you know.

Now that I clarified the waters regarding who in a limited scale of human interactions is, I believe that everyone will think thoroughly the answer to the question of how do your relate to other employees in your company/division/group.

FyI, the answer I was looking for was something like…"my colleagues are very knowledgeable, we share responsibilities in a matrix environment following strict procedures, and provide for support to other divisions as a group…we interact in a very positive manner, and resolve conflicts immediately to allow proper workflow…", and then I would ask for examples of responsibility sharing, external support and conflict resolution. When he used the word friend, the conversation departed. The interview lost essence as of qualifying the individual for a job, but trying to understand how this individual relates to other people.

I hope these insights help you provide great answers in your job interview, and further enable you getting that ideal job, and also to shed more light on the relations you have with the people that surrounds you. Knowing who falls under which category, will also allow you setup the right expectations.

Originally published on March 29, 2015

Getting Inspired to Make Your Job and Life Better

Today, I am not going to discuss about Clinical Research in particular, but about all of us as a multidimensional individuals. To understand how we can get inspired to be better and more productive, hence happier, we have to understand our different dimensions. One of our dimensions is who we are in our private life, the second, who we are at our work and profession, the third what people perceive of who we are, and the last, of what we perceive about ourselves.

What are the sources of inspiration that drives our creativity and willingness to get on with our lives every day?

Self confidence and assertiveness is based initially on our perception of ourselves and supported by how other people perceive us. However, we may be perceived as two completely different persons, one at work (or outside of our house) and the other at home. Further, we may give others a completely different impression of ourselves and also we can have a different picture of ourselves compared to what others perceive and how we are perceived at home and at work. This seem to be like a personality disorder with 4 different personalities in one person but is not. Is the norm. We are the same person, what differentiates us from one dimension to the other is the environment we are and the people around us. Regardless of the dimension our life takes at a give time, the sources of inspiration are going to be the same, and the change due to our ability to get inspired is going to be observed in every dimension.

The question here is how we can get inspired to be better in our job and life. You cannot be better just because, you have to have a reason, a "je nai sais quoi" to get to the next level.

Inspiration is what make things to improve, inspiration drives creativity and invention.

What are the sources of inspiration, your muse, that drives our creativity and willingness to get on with our lives every day?

Depending on your personality and ambitions, the muse is different for different people.

Consider that you have to wake up every morning to go to work, besides the need to earn a living, what does drive you to do it? why that particular job?

We all have a reason in our lives that keeps us going, however, few of us are lucky enough to be inspired by a muse to make things better. But once we find her, our creativity and imagination take us to incredible achievements in all dimensions of our lives.

Inspiration is what make things to improve, inspiration drives creativity and invention.

As a manager, and also a parent, I am constantly motivating people to do things, to bring new ideas, to invent, to be the first to do something. However, motivating is not enough until they get inspired. I had cases where people who were very motivated to work but did not know what to do better or how. There is where a muse comes very handy.

All of us, as the great artists and scientist, have a muse. The issue is that many of us have not found her yet.

To find your source of inspiration, you have to be true to yourself, your abilities and qualities. Your image of yourself has to be a positive one. Your self-confidence and assertiveness have to be positioned in a positive mode. Creativity is always positive and contribute to the general good. Being creative can never be detrimental, otherwise is not creative, but the opposite, destructive.

Every morning, when I wake up, I first think on the reasons I have to wake up, then what my responsibilities are that day, then what can be improved, and at the end I look up to my muse to give me the inspiration I need to be creative and make things better for everyone.

> *"Creativity is always positive and contribute to the general good. Being creative can never be detrimental, otherwise is not creative, but the opposite, destructive"*

Some people find their muse in religion, others in art, or nature. Some never find her, because are too busy thinking on what others think about them.

What is your muse? do you consider you can drive creativity and invention? Do you think you can improve things at work or in your personal life if only you get that drive...call it "inspiration"....

Originally published on April 26, 2015

Clinical Research Training Accessibility

"Training and education is one of the largest benefits an employee can have while working for a company"

Clinical research professionals have to continuously get training and education to remain updated on all changes in regulations and to further ensure compliance and guarantee the quality of their job.

Although companies provide for limited training and education, presently a vast majority of clinical research associates (CRAs) are contractors that do not qualify for company sponsored training and education. That leaves a large group of professionals (mostly monitors) that are responsible to ensure that patients are safe, and that studies are done in compliance with the protocol without the needed training and education.

"without proper training you will not be able to advance in your clinical research career, nor become up to date with the constant changes in the industry and regulations"

It is important to highlight that training and education is one of the largest benefits an employee can have while working for a company.

The majority of the in-class training programs for clinical research (CR) professionals are very expensive, and only large companies can afford. Also, they require days at a time for off-site training, what implies the added travel and accommodation expenses

Individuals as well as smaller companies are limited on the access to proper training and education to do their job due to 2 factors,

- one is affordability and
- the other accessibility.

Affordability is only one part of the equation, especially for contractors who need to improve their skills to remain competitive in the market. However, affordability is not the only issue, accessibility also is. You may be asking yourself why accessibility? because not everyone can put aside 2-3 days in a given period of time to dedicate exclusively to training when they are paid for the hours they effectively do their job. To determine what would make a win-win situation to deliver high quality affordable and accessible CR education we assisted in a survey of almost 500 professionals to determine which type of educational delivery system they prefer and the length of time they were willing to dedicate to training at a given time. The results surprised me, because the majority (regardless of age, experience and gender) preferred web-based training, and were willing to dedicate between 1-4 hours to training at a given time. Therefore, the results of the survey allow me to say that the majority of professionals now would prefer web-based training programs (e.g.e-courses) and that is not more than 4 hours in length total.

With the introduction of excellent software-free web-based solutions to education, and the advancement of technology and accessibility to internet, more companies and individuals are turning to web-based e-Learning solutions to meet their needs.

Those solutions allow participants to:

- train at their own pace
- review and repeat lessons
- test their knowledge though interactive tools
- blog (interact with peers)
- interact with the instructor (on-line and off-line)
- and become certified

Many companies offer web-based programs, however not all those programs engage the audience towards learning, but mostly provide an informative approach. Therefore, if you are a contractor, or want to improve your qualifications, or are assigned to choose a good training solution for your company, you must do your research of web-based clinical research training, see the options available and whether the delivery format is good for you.

To choose a Web-based training programs, you have to look into

- how good and concise they are (straight to the point of discussion)
- what type of training solution is (e-course, webinar, web-meeting, webcast, etc.)
- is it synchronous (you have to be there at a given time) or asynchronous (on your own time)
- what is the quality of the presentation (how does it look and sounds like, try a test version)
- does it have instructors presenting or professional actors?
- does it allow participants get in touch with the instructors?

- are there discussion boards or blogs to further discuss with peers? and
- is it affordable and accessible at any time?

If you have any insights, please comment, I would like to hear from you!

Originally published on April 21, 2015

Do Not Get Caught with Your Pants Down in a Job Interview

I choose this title, because that's what it is "Do not get caught with your pants down in a job interview"!!! I will be discussing real situations from my experience interviewing people, where potential candidates burned their bridges before they even got a chance at getting properly interviewed.

Although this applies to all potential candidates to any job, I am giving examples that are related to clinical research, since that was where my experience comes from interviewing hundreds of candidates from entry to senior levels.

First, a phone job interview is only the first step into the candidate selection process. Depending on the industry, the type of job, position level, and specialized knowledge, the approach may vary. You may go though many stages of the interviewing process or only one. Larger companies have a complete procedure you will go trough, while smaller companies will rely only on the face to face job interview.

When you decided to apply for a particular job, you may have given lots of consideration and asked yourself: (or not)

- do I have the qualifications?
- is my experience enough?
- does my education limits my ability to apply?
- am I prepared to travel a lot?
- would I relocate?
- would I work in a contract or permanent basis?

Regardless the reasons why are you applying for a particular job (mind you many people try to apply to jobs they are not qualified for just to give it a chance, DO NOT DO THAT! unless you know what your are talking about and what are you getting into), you are going to send your resume and a cover letter, and expect for a feed back. You may have applied like this for tens of jobs. You lost count already...

And then one day (may be months after you applied) the phone rings.....(actually the cellphone because that was the only number you provided for). Let's look at the conversation:

Company: Hello, I am Joan Smith from XYZ pharmaceutical company, and I am calling in response to your job application for a position within our clinical group. Is this a good time for you to talk?

You: Hmm...oh, ok. sure. (in the back of your mind you are thinking "what is the job I applied for?, I do not remember sending an application?, what did I say in my cover letter? or my resume?)

Company: Great, let me ask you for how many years have you been monitoring clinical trials?

You: well, several years (you know at that moment this is for a monitoring job but....oh gosh, I do not remember what I wrote to make sure it fits the requirement) -in the background she can hear your dog barking and your kid just flushed the toilet-

Company: Hmmm.. You also wrote in you resume that you have experience dealing with FDA-GCP inspections. How many did you have to deal with in a typical year?

You: Well, you know...they were so many that I cannot tell you from the top of my head... a number...may be 8 or 10? .....

Company: Good. Thank you for your time. We will send you an email with the next steps. Good Bye.

You got caught with your pants down!!!

Although the phone pre-screening is a typical approach many companies utilize to weed out applicants. You have failed all three questions. Let's dissect the 45 second conversation.

First, you were not prepared to take that call regardless of the position they were calling about. For a phone interview you have to be prepared and make sure that your state of mind is setup to respond sharply.

Your response to the first question should have been ..." I am tied up right now, can you give me your number, I will call you back in 5 minutes or tomorrow morning, or call me back in 5 minutes or tomorrow at x hours"... Then prepare yourself for the drill. You must be in a quiet place, with no background noise and distractions. It is your FIRST IMPRESSION and the only one for that position.

Then, when the phone interview started again, you should have asked..."I believe you are calling me for the position of Sr. CRA I applied in May..." that puts you in the same page and lets them know that you are prepared to answer the questions.

Second, when she said..."let me ask you for how many years have you been monitoring clinical trials?"... your answer..."several years..." speaks loudly that you really do not have the experience they are looking for but are here for a try, several lets you be in the range of more than two but less than 10. Although that by itself may not completely disqualify you, it is a minus.

Then, the following question was the checkmate one. She directly asked you a very specific question that tests not only your experience but your knowledge about regulatory processes and procedures and that was..."You also wrote in you resume that you have experience dealing with FDA-GCP inspections. How many did you have to deal with in a typical year?. You said nonchalantly 8-10 inspections, in an asking tone. (FyI, the FDA conducts a total of about 600 inspections per year, targeting only 2% of sites/sponsors/CROs maximum, what means that you had a probability to be inspected at the most once every year, mind you there some sites/sponsors and CRO's that are targeted more often but that is because they run a lot of studies or had observations in previous inspections).

She got you with your pants down! you were not straight forward with your experience. You may have been involved in an inspection only once, and you should have made the most out of that experience during the interview rather than answering with a number.

You lost your opportunity to get to the next step of the selection process because,

- you were not prepared,
- you overestimated your experience, and
- you did not handle the questions properly.

Originally published on April 25, 2015

The Ancient Clinical Research Process

Imagine yourself today, in the 21st century, building a power plant producing DC (direct current) electricity to power a city, or riding a horse to work, or better, doing the laundry on the Hudson River. Why not? Our families did that in the recent past. Oh, I have better one, using the abacus to calculate the maximum load for a steel beam. For decades that was the best way of doing things, absolutely acceptable and in most cases the norm, let's call it, the gold standard. Of course, we would not be doing that now that we have more refined and efficient (not really very fuel efficient) methods.

When we look into how we are developing new therapeutic products, we are doing just that. We are testing and testing and testing (trying), until we prove ourselves that either it may work or not, or we do not really know it since for the sake of bringing something to the market we assumed too much. We are using a method that yield a failed product in more than 85% of the cases. Nonetheless, we still keep using it and just wanting more and more. It seems like the parody of the crazy man, who repeats the same thing time and time again expecting for the outcome to differ, like "one day it will really work".

We are using a method that yield a failed product in more than 85% of the cases.

Why the clinical research process cannot be sustainable anymore?

We invested billions in technology, we are able to collect an enormous amount of data directly from patients into databases with minimal human intervention, hence less errors. We were able to satisfy the statisticians' need of very large sample sizes and faster enrollment with globalization of studies to prove or disprove hypotheses, mainly based on assumptions that skew our ability of interpretation, being the biggest one, in which all subjects "behave" normally (will respond statistically normal between 1 or better 2 standard deviations). And yet the reality is that we did not have a real breakthrough, actually most of the drugs developed are more of the same, with a twist. That twist seems to be sufficient enough to convince most that it is something new and different. Everyone wants to be in the business of clinical research, mind you that is the only business that has more than 85% failure rate after $ 2.5 BN of investment. Of course, if a drug proves to make a difference, according to pre-established criteria defined in the protocols, then Jackpot!!!

It's all a matter of perception

Actually, I perceive the drug development process as shooting into the air, very up high, and expecting that a duck will fall. Most of the times, actually 85% of the time, nothing happens, sometimes we catch a pigeon or a sparrow, may be in the best case scenario we catch swan or a stork (little use because they are not really edible, but can do), while looking for a blockbuster. However, we never catch a cow or a pig (the real new drug, the blockbuster). Why? Because they DO NOT FLY! What do I mean with all this? That it is the same with clinical trials, we do not have major breakthroughs because we are aiming in the wrong direction, using the wrong tools, and we do not really know what to expect at the end.

However, at a staggering cost of developing a new drug of up to U$S 2.5 billion and growing as I speak, it makes the clinical research business enterprise unsustainable.

Consequently, we have to leave the horse and get a car, switch to AC, use a good washer and leave the abacus. What do I mean with that? I mean, a real paradigm shift has to happen to the Clinical Research process,to be able to really bring new therapeutic innovations that are going to be meaningful, not only financially but medically and to humanity.

> *"at a staggering cost of developing a new drug of up to U$S 2.5 billion and growing as I speak, it makes the clinical research business enterprise unsustainable"*

Let's analyze the clinical research picture (just a few for example purposes):

- It takes an average of 12.5 years to put a new drug in the market, and that did not improve at all in 25 years despite huge investments.
- Just really few new drugs (that either address unmet needs or a previously controlled condition, but in a different way) are approved every year.
- Many new drugs are not efficient in the market as proposed during development
- Many drugs have safety concerns when they reach the market
- Data transparency seems to be a never-ending ritual of becoming

- In time, while the cost of development increases, the number of new drugs per dollar invested decreases

Information technology (IT) did not make the great impact in data flow as expected to allow new and better drugs to reach the market faster, but only to achieve failure a little earlier. From the experience we have now, I can venture to say that IT only allowed increase the burden of data and patients in a clinical trial, actually permitting mega studies, hence increasing the cost of development. This makes the perceived return on investment on IT very questionable. Nevertheless, IT is a necessary tool that aimed at the right direction, it can improve and reinvent the clinical research enterprise.

The gold standard for clinical research is the randomized placebo controlled clinical trial, shouldn't we do better than that?

Previous attempts at changes in paradigm did not improve the process today, whereas for example adaptive design may encounter many statistical challenges, or faster road-maps to market in early development may open a can of worm (holes).

Even as I write, the "Risk Based Monitoring" approach, to be amended in GCP/ICH has taken the form of great advancement with a focus on "quality systems" and increased standardization of processes. However, the clinical research paradigm remains the same.

Originally published on April 29, 2015

The One Mistake in Perception of Drug Efficacy vs. Efficiency

In controlled clinical trials, we always measure drug EFFICACY, whereas we measure discrete variables in a very limited patient population homogeneous enough to consider certain variables that may affect the outcome as constant, and assume that the outcome or difference encountered is due to the therapeutic intervention.

The sample of study represents only a minimal fraction of the real market population for the particular indication. In general, the inclusion/exclusion criteria regardless of the fact that selects subjects based on characteristics that they must share from the diagnostic, prophylactic and disease history as well as phenotypic and sometimes genotypic point of view, also introduces bias to the sample since it is not a random sample of the population, but a skewed one. This is what I call in my book "the biased sample" in clinical trials. This means that the results also are going to be skewed, in which the efficacy observed (if any) depends on the criteria for measurement and is going to be in function of the particular selected population, and does not intend to represent the general population for the indication.

The sample of study represents only a minimal fraction of the real market population for the particular indication....it is not a random sample of the population, but a skewed one.

The criteria for measurement in clinical trials

It seems that there is a misinterpretation about what does it means that a drug product is efficacious from the point of view of its development targets.

Being efficacious means that it met a specified criterion from the statistical point of view where we were able to see a true difference between groups in function of a variable of study, let call it the efficacy variable. That true difference, although real, may not represent a breakthrough in medicine, but just that the product met a target criterion in a very specific population (e.g. reduce BP levels by 5% in moderate hypertense patients without any other underlying condition and not taking any other medication and where the BMI was between normal to 4% above normal values).

Being efficacious means that it met a specified criterion from the statistical point of view where we were able to see a true difference between groups in function of a variable of study, let call it the efficacy variable.

As development progresses, some of the criteria is more relaxed to increase (theoretically) the level of heterogeneity. The age group is going to be the same (between 18-65 years for instance). As the case I present as example now patients taking some medication are allowed in the studies (with concomitant medications to treat inter-current illnesses), however medications related to any cardiovascular condition might be excluded –including diuretics- as well as may be anti anxiety and other CNS drugs. Again, the patient population enrolled as the sample will be in the younger range since they are healthier taking less medications, and again we will have a bias entered in the study in which the sample is skewed towards less compromised subjects. Now is where multi-centre/multi country studies are necessary to be able to find the required number of those patients that are moderate hypertense, within a normal BMI, otherwise healthy and may be taking medication for unrelated conditions as allergies, gastric reflux, acidity, and supplements, because they are the very few in one region. (many of my investigators complain regularly saying..."where do I find those patients?"..).

Once the development is completed with such type of patients in a sample size large enough, and selected from a variety of sources and geographical locations, where we continue observing the target efficacy outcome as true, we consider that the drug is efficacious enough to pursue marketing. Let's assume that there are no safety concerns to worry about.

We are approved! A new drug reaches the market!

The marketing teams of the pharmaceutical company is in full action following approval, selling the new drug with all the information provided by the clinical development/regulatory teams in regards of safety and efficacy. Phrases like ..."the product safety profile does not differ from similar drugs already in the market"... or ..."no safety concerns were identified during development"... fills the marketing materials.

Also, for efficacy the drug is going to represented as..."in clinical trials a real 5 % reduction in BP was observed after the first dose, and a further 10% after subsequent doses"...and that is generally true. However, there are footnotes to the words that directs to papers, or SmPCs (Summary of Product Characteristics) or other supporting publications where it explains that the outcome, as described was observed in patients 18-35 years of age that they were the bulk of the subjects providing data, while older (36-55 years) had a more modest reduction, and for 56-65 there was not enough data to say that the percentage reduction is statistically significant. Although the marketing pamphlet does not indicate that fact directly, the references do but are seldom read by the prescribing physician. (remember this is a hypothetical scenario and does not represent any real case).

The Efficiency Surprise

The drug marketing is in full swing, it is selling very well in response to the marketing excitement and the option of having a better alternative. However, results in the clinic seem minimal, patients return to the doctor very soon with BP uncontrolled, and other drugs are being added to control hypertension. May be a diuretic goes first, and then an ACE inhibitor.

The drug EFFICIENCY is not as expected. The responses observed in the clinic are mixed, resorting back to the old approach of poly-therapy. At this point the doctor does not know exactly which drug is the best of the prescribed, and assumes a synergistic effect, that may be possible. As the marketing swing continues, so the drug sales.

The issue here is that although the drug was not misrepresented from the point of view of efficacy in clinical trials, the prescribing physician assumed that the efficacy is extrapolable to efficiency in the clinic. Therefore, the lack of reading the supporting material to the marketing approach to determine exactly the population of study, are responsible for the assumption that efficacy and efficiency are the same thing.

"the prescribing physician assumed that the efficacy is extrapolable to efficiency in the clinic."

In this example, that is only hypothetical and does not reflect any drug in the market in particular, I tried in a very simplistic manner to show the difference between EFFICACY in clinical trials and EFFICIENCY in the market.

Originally published May 1, 2015

The Placebo Effect May Invalidate Our Assumptions

Just recently, I was discussing about misconceptions regarding efficacy of a drug demonstrated in clinical trials and its efficiency in the clinic. The fact that it did not draw attention with comments or rebuttals just proves that the confusion is still ongoing.

Also, just a couple of days back I was trying to start a conversation regarding the clinical trial process and the shortcomings we are observing as mostly responsible for increasing the cost of development and reducing the chances to find really good therapeutic product. It seems that there is limitation in the awareness of the clinical trial process as an enterprise that, as a whole discipline, is little understood by the key players.

I hope that this article today, raises some great feedback, because it touches the very nerve of the clinical trial process, its "gold standard", the randomized placebo-controlled study.

In the quest to determine whether a therapeutic product is really responsible for the difference in observed response, comparison to placebo and other active treatments is the norm. Further, the establishment of the superiority to placebo and/or controls may hold the key to potential approval.

But, what does it mean the comparison to placebo? Let's look at the placebo itself first.

The placebo effect was described a long time ago as a nonspecific positive response to a "sugar pill" driven mostly by patient's perception that they are being treated. Although these are pure placebos, the ones utilized in clinical trials are non-pure placebos because they contain substances not considered pharmacologically active and are devoid of the active ingredient of study.

The placebo effect is very well observed in certain conditions, in others, like malignancies, infections, and infestations, is rarer. In an early study in 1955 it was demonstrated that about 35% of patients treated with placebo do respond positively to treatment (with some exceptions regarding the condition), especially in clinical trials for psychiatric conditions like anxiety and depression where the numbers may be even higher.

The placebo effect was described a long time ago as a nonspecific positive response to a "sugar pill" driven mostly by patient's perception that they are being treated.

Why should we be concerned about the placebo effect?

Very simple, because it is an observed and very real effect, with tangible outcomes, and that may produce the desired responses without the safety issues observed in "active substances".

> *"the (...placebos...) utilized in clinical trials are non-pure placebos because they contain substances not considered pharmacologically active and are (only) devoid of the active ingredient of study"*

Fortunately, there is active interest in the study of the placebo effect and recently the program Placebo Studies & Therapeutic Encounter (PiPS) was initiated by the Beth Israel Deaconess Medical Center / Harvard Medical School to study the effect in guidance, practice and patient choice on the use of placebos. Dr. Ted Kaptchuck is the leader of the program, and in a forum conducted on December 9, 2013, very important elements were discussed regarding the use of placebos that support the concern about the perception of the placebo role in clinical research.

> *"it was demonstrated that about 35% of patients treated with placebo do respond positively to treatment"*

The first point I want to make is: should we discard a drug because is not better than placebo?

Dr. Michael J Barry explained in the forum that in a study conducted to demonstrate the efficacy of Saw Palmetto in controlling urinary symptoms in men, observed that the Saw Palmetto arm was not different than placebo. Nevertheless, a tangible beneficial effect was observed, and it increased with time and dose. Of course, the right conclusion is that in controlled clinical trials, Saw Palmetto did not fare better than placebo. But that did not mean that a clinical meaningful effect was not observed, only that is not different than placebo. Further, when Dr. Harold C. Sox brought up the data of the no treatment arm, both placebo and Saw Palmetto made a clinically significant difference. Therefore, the effect is very real, and has tangible outcomes. Then, what does it means from the therapeutic point of view? Should we consider placebo a treatment option for the above condition when a clinically meaningful response is observed?

What do we make about the placebo effect in comparison to active substances?

In my opinion, the placebo effect should be considered as a very important response to perceived intervention, with minimal adverse events, and with large therapeutic perspective if demonstrated further in specific clinical trials for that purpose.

It is time to understand that placebo effect is not an "inconvenience" in clinical trials that masks the effect of potential therapeutic products, but a tool for practicing physicians to address medical issues in a less aggressive manner. Dr. Russell S. Phillips, in that very same forum explained that there is no guidance available for the use of placebos in the clinic, and that it might be another tool for treatment. The lack of clinical trials to demonstrate the potential benefits of using placebos in specific conditions, limits the ability of prescribing physicians to effectively rely on its use, and be perceived as providing deceptive treatment.

It may be that, as explained by Dr. Sox, the placebo effect may be at least in part responsible for the effects that we observe in drugs, and that the drug effect is a sum of the biochemical effect of the active ingredient in the drug itself and the placebo effect with an unknown pathway.

Shouldn't placebo therefore be considered an "active substance" by virtue of response?

Furthermore, there are studies demonstrating that when placebo acupuncture is delivered in an empathetic manner, the clinical response is significantly greater, so what this means now? Is empathy itself stimuli enough to promote or enhance response to treatment? We should not forget the very evidence that newborns thrive better when cuddled and handled, than left without physical contact (is this an innate response to ensure survival?)

May be in this way we can explain why certain clinical trial sites have better objective responses than in others, just by virtue of patient approach. In globally dispersed clinical trial sites, there might be the unknown or not addressed bias introduced due to "cultural" patient management. In this case, if the sample is unbalanced in size per site or geographical location (keep in mind that some studies provide most of the submission data from one country or one geographical region, with good analysis of interference on the response driven by site specific interactions), regardless of the analysis of site specific interactions on the response, that particular aspect (empathy and perception of treatment) may play a role in response without being considered an interference factor but part of the response itself (embedded in such manner that cannot be statistically differentiated).

It is my opinion that:

Clinical trials should be more critical regarding the placebo effect itself, and that placebo vs. no intervention (from historical data or baseline data) should be analysed first, to determine whether the placebo effect is sufficient enough to classify it as clinically significant, and then therapeutically permissive.

Clinical Trial sites should be standardized as to treatment approach to patient to minimize the "empathy effect" on outcomes

Also, we should be conducting long term studies to determine the sustainability of the placebo effects on indications where it is clinically significant.

Placebo effect may act synergistically with drugs enhancing its effects and therefore when we only observe a true difference, it might be by virtue of perception of intervention.

Another important thing we should be looking into is whether certain drugs that may affect our perceptions, feelings, and mental state in order to revert the placebo effect or even eliminate it yielding well established treatments otherwise efficacious, useless.

It is also important to realize that many drugs in the market have very well-defined effect, irreverent of a placebo response, measured directly and where the effect is linear to response in function of the dose (within a range). That is a fact. However, in other drugs the effect is limited, subject to long term treatment, where the reassurance of potential effect by the part of the prescribing physician might eventually take the form of an expected response, nevertheless is a placebo effect.

Originally published on May 3, 2015

7 Reasons Why More Than 85% of Investigational Drugs Fail

The clinical stage of the drug development process is very complex with extremely complicated protocols, tight timelines, cost overruns and high expectations. Have you ever thought why the failure rate is more than 85% in some cases?

We ask that question ourselves all the time. For the last 20 years, I am studying the reason why the clinical research process is not living up to their expectations, being a high-risk investment with returns limited by the patent protections and enforcement of patent rights. There is not simple answer to this question, maybe we have many unknowns and few equations. We seem helpless, unable to solve the issues and confined in a regulatory and systemic box.

Although I do not intend to discuss about the failures of the clinical research process per se, I will discuss 7 of the most common mistakes that prompt rapid failure, as identified.

The clinical stage of the drug development process is very complex with extremely complicated protocols, tight timelines, cost overruns and high expectations. Have you ever thought why the failure rate is more than 85% in some cases?

Mistake #1

The wrong indication

Once the pre-clinical development is completed, and there is a reasonable evidence that the product might be safe and have therapeutic purpose in humans, the biggest question is, which indication the product should be developed for? The answer to the question is going to be influenced by the aim to develop a product within highly profitable indications (preferred by sponsor companies), market size and competition. Therefore, of several potential indications possible for a potential therapeutic product, the most profitable ones are going to be favoured. Those indications are going to be pursued, and not necessarily the ones with higher probability of success. Of course, there is no sense on developing drugs that are not perceived as a good ROI (return on investment), what is reasonable. This is one of the points where science and business intersects. Therefore, the selection of the indication plays a key role in the success of the product developed. Simply, if we choose the wrong indication, we are not going to see the responses we expect, and the product fails early.

"the selection of the indication plays a key role in the success of the product developed"

Mistake #2

The wrong dose or dose range

Once the indication is selected, we have to run dose finding studies to determine which the range of doses is where the product works the best. Those doses must be well below the maximum tolerated in humans to be practical and should allow dose adjustments to control response. The kinetics of dose vs response should be linear, and measurable by accepted methods. Many times, sponsors to be within a safety zone, work with doses well below the minimum effective dose, or sometimes the entire development is done in within a dose range that does not satisfy the efficacy outcomes sought, and therefore the product fails to meet the development objectives.

Many times, sponsors to be within a safety zone, work with doses well below the minimum effective dose... that does not satisfy the efficacy outcomes sought.

Mistake #3

Efficacy endpoints overrated

Of course, to make it to the market you have to demonstrate that your product really makes a difference compared, not only to placebo, but to the active comparators. The point here is that sponsors tend to develop drugs that have already established a track record (e.g. a new statin), is like a safety net because the efficacy of statins is already proved historically. However, targeting the same molecular pathway may not render the product more efficacious (if that is sought), but just will allow you tap on the spot. Trying to demonstrate that your product is better from the efficacy stand point (while being more of the same) it might backfire, despite being safe and efficacious as comparable products in the market, it does not live up to the expectation of being an X % better than…

Other way of seeing this point is when we seek a considerable difference between our product and the competition to make the investigational product a potential "blockbuster" since the ROI we seek is too large for what the market has to offer. Well, setting the bar too high may be the most sorrowful source of failure.

> *...setting the bar too high may be the most sorrowful source of failure...*

Mistake #4

Serious Safety Concerns previously underestimated

Regardless of all the precautions and analysis conducted in preclinical and in phase I, the product has demonstrated to have a benefit/risk ratio that is unacceptable within the dose ranges where a desirable efficacy response is observed. Then, this is the end of the product. However, where the mistake is? Well, the mistake is in the first sentence, I mean....did you really estimated the risk properly? Did you undermined animal safety data in lieu of spices specificity or that you could not replicate the effect in other animals? Were some safety indicators overlooked?

May be answering to those questions will allow you avoid costly failures in the middle of clinical development in the future.

Mistake #5

Wrong patient population

The inclusion/ exclusion criteria.... With the aim to select a homogeneous subject population who will 'safely' respond to the drug and have the condition for which the drug is being developed, we may end up selecting the very same wrong subjects for which the drug may not work at all. Or the criteria may be so stringent, that investigators enrol the closest, but not really the subjects with the indication we are looking for. Then, if they do not have the condition, they will not respond to it. Very simple, eh?

That is why the subject selection criteria plays a definite role in the success of a product within an indication (after the indication itself). In the extremely complicated protocols we have now, that criteria become one of the major hurdles for enrollment and subsequent success of a study. We have grown from an average 10 criteria for inclusion/exclusion, to more than 40. Remember that the sample has to exist in the real world too, otherwise you will eventually fail in the post marketing phase….

"(inclusion/exclusion) criteria become one of the major hurdles for enrollment and subsequent success of a study"

Mistake #6

Underestimated Manufacturing, or Intrinsic Product Costs

Although this is not a mistake from the clinical standpoint, sometimes the source of failure is nothing more than manufacturing processes that were underestimated at the bench level, and when the manufacturing process had to be scaled up, it could not be efficiently replicated. The intrinsic product costs have to do with the physico-chemical properties of the product itself that makes it very unstable, with a limited shelf life, or the yield of the active ingredient due to its stereochemical nature is very small in which only one isomer is active and the other…toxic…etc. Those are issues that should have played a role during product development, before large investments were made in clinical development.

Mistake #7

Marketing concerns

Under or overestimating market size for the product (that will be limited by the indication and the patient population eligible to use it), as well as market competition, it is a source of failure in clinical development. Marketing will push for a wider base population in clinical development, to increase the market size, and then, the product cannot live up to that expectation. With a smaller market base, regardless of high efficacy and good safety, a product will not make it to the market because the market base does not make business sense. (This is another point where business and science intersects).

Marketing will push for a wider base population in clinical development, to increase the market size, and then, the product cannot live up to that expectation (failing in efficacy and/or safety)

Do you see these mistakes in your daily work? Do you consider them relevant to what you do?, which other mistakes would you add?

Originally published on May 15, 2015

Clinical Research in a Globally Diverse Population

Clinical trials are evolving towards a more complex and costly endeavor where sample sizes are increasing in lieu of satisfying the statistical method established to determine if a difference exists and if that is clinically significant and market sensible. We have been witnesses of cost increases in the order of 10-25% annually since the inception of Good Clinical Practices. On the other hand, timeliness to bring a product to the market are longer, and the clinical research business enterprise is at its lowest with a less than 20% success rate from bench to shelf.

Here I am going to mention only 10 reasons why we need to satisfy the ever-increasing need for more patients.

1. More stringent inclusion/exclusion criteria that makes the ideal patient for the study limited
2. More outcome measures
3. Very high level of complexity of the study design that deters investigators and patients
4. Cost containment

5. Investigators attrition due to increased liability in the FDA region
6. Regulatory pressure on the design
7. Increased competition and heightened biosimilar development projects
8. Limited product innovation prompting increased number of studies to establish potential candidates
9. Shift from personalized medicine to precision medicine?
10. Shrinking timeliness

We have been witnesses of cost increases in the order of 10-25% annually since the inception of Good Clinical Practices

However, a reasonable observation steers towards the issue of variability in the populations utilized that impact the clinical trial outcomes in such extent that the results are not encouraging, hence feeding failure. Statistical considerations include the issue of patient variability, but only to a limited extent. I am going to present only briefly 15 sources of variability in clinical trials that are mainly geographically based, some of which are included in the analysis while others are considered normal:

1. Access to regular health care
2. Health culture
3. Regional standard of medical practice
4. Diet and religion
5. Diet and customs
6. Genetics
7. Epigenetics
8. Natural environmental factors (high altitudes, proximity to sea/rivers/mountains, extreme cold/hot weather)
9. Artificial environmental factors (exposure to toxic substances –smog, toxic fumes- exposure to drug metabolites in the drinking water, radiation, EMF?)
10. Wars, displacement, re adaptation

11. Racial factors that influence health (Mediterranean, Latino, Scandinavian, Slovene, Asian, South-asian, African, etc)
12. Other medical paradigms utilized concurrently but seldom reported (Chinese medicine, Ayurveda, Homeopathic, Aboriginal medicine, Herbal remedies and teas)
13. Stress and culture
14. Regionally based Inter-current illnesses (diagnosed and un-diagnosed)
15. Access to technology, internet, smartphones

Now is up to you to determine if these are valid, and if you have other factors that may influence, and you consider them as important.

Originally published on June 14, 2015

Biotrial Phase I study and the death of a healthy volunteer

On January 15, 2016, all over the news we could read about the "accident". The BBC reported that ..."One man is brain-dead and another five people are in hospital after an experimental drug was administered to 90 people in a French clinical trial". Although I do not prefer Wikipedia as my source of information, they reported that ..."In 2016, Bial commissioned a contract research organization to run a phase one clinical trial for BIA 10-2474, an FAAH (Fatty acid amide hydrolase) inhibitor that targets the endocannabinoid system. Testing of the drug in Rennes resulted in hospitalisations of six subjects receiving the drug, with one becoming brain dead"...

On Sunday, January 17, 2016, almost one week after being hospitalized, one of the healthy volunteers who suffered a catastrophic adverse event, has died. The BBC reports that "...a man left brain-dead after an experimental drug trial in France has died, local media report"...

Actually, the core of my post is not to discuss about the investigational drug, or the companies involved in the worst case scenario of clinical research. I understand that they followed rules, regulations and the protocol. Nevertheless, I want to bring awareness of what does it mean a catastrophic adverse event in phase I clinical development, fast tracking research, and start the conversation regarding healthy volunteers in clinical research.

First, let's talk about catastrophic adverse events. A catastrophic adverse event is what we call a serious unexpected adverse drug reaction. This type of event can cause death or is so severe that can incapacitate the healthy subject, in this case, for life. Catastrophic adverse events, by nature can be irreversible, and may produce life-long lasting effects. In this case, death was the outcome for one healthy man. The BBC reports that "...The hospital said the other five remained in a stable condition - four had "neurological problems" and the fifth had no symptoms..."

Next, phase I clinical research, per se, conducted generally in healthy volunteers, is not free from controversy from the ethical and moral standpoint, but somehow precluded by the version of October 2013 of the "declaration of Helsinki" , where states that "...research on patients or healthy volunteers requires the supervision of a competent and appropriately qualified physician or other health care professional"... Actually, the original version of 1964 dedicates an entire heading to non-therapeutic medical research, in which, ..."In research on man, the interest of science and society should never take precedence over considerations related to the well-being of the subject"... That section was completely eliminated in the newer versions. Not having an explicit section dedicated to the protection of healthy volunteers in clinical research embedded into the declaration, that is the foundation of Good Clinical Practices, might have permitted the streamlined approval and conduct of phase I clinical trials. At the end of the day, as the declaration states..." Medical progress is based on research that ultimately must include studies involving human subjects"...

James Gallagher, health editor, BBC News website writes that "...this is the bitter price of the new medicines we take for granted. Testing such experimental drugs, at the cutting edge of science, can never be completely risk-free...". With all the respect that deserves such a great editor, I beg to disagree. The "accident" was nothing more that the resultant of lack of ethical and scientific basis for the inclusion of healthy volunteers in phase I studies in order to obtain clean data regarding pharmacokinetics and safety of an investigational drug without the interference of disease and concomitant medications. In my opinion, Phase I safety and pharmacokinetics studies in healthy volunteers will not produce better or cleaner data than studies in patient volunteers. It will only provide for "nicer" data. Consequently, only the healthy subject who was the one suffering such an event paid the ultimate price for the betterment of humanity. However, we have to keep in mind that (let me repeat myself) ..."In research on man, the interest of science and society should never take precedence over considerations related to the well-being of the subject"... Furthermore, Claude Bernard expressed that "... one should not injure one person regardless of the benefits that might come to others..." In addition, the Belmont Report establishes that"...The problem posed by these imperatives (Do not do harm, and to benefit patients according to doctor's best judgement) is to decide when it is justifiable to seek certain benefits despite the risks involved, and when the benefits should be foregone because of the risks..."

Lastly, I want to highlight the concept of fast tracking in clinical research, involving large amount of subjects in very complicated studies, very early in development, with an oversight based on risk. It is important at this point to contemplate the issue of wanting to get to the market very fast, without having collected enough safety information in a progressive manner that can increase the confidence of the physician and the subject. It is seldom recommended that phase one, healthy volunteer studies are conducted in large samples. Generally, samples sizes are quite small, and exposure to the investigation product is gradual with interim safety analyses between escalations of dose.

In conclusion, in my opinion, the "accident" as referred to in all news outlets regarding the catastrophic adverse events in a phase I study, is the resultant of a pragmatic approach to clinical research based on ethical considerations that does not include special provisions for the inclusion of healthy volunteers.

Now that I started the conversation, I will be very glad to hear your opinion about the topic.

Originally published on January 15, 2016

Where are the clinical research jobs?

Background analysis

Clinical research as a business enterprise has evolved greatly in the last 20 years. Rules, regulations and international guidelines have been developed and further adjusted to the new technologies and advances in data collection and handling.

> *"personalized medicine...data driven approach to care... to real time data acquisition, analysis and reporting...change(d)... the scope of work and job descriptions of one of the key figures in clinical research: the monitors or clinical research associates"*

From a general approach to "one size (dose) fits most" we evolved to "personalized medicine" and "patient centered care". As medicine itself changed to a data driven approach to care, drug development also steered to real time data acquisition, analysis and reporting. All this had to be accompanied by a change in the scope of work and job descriptions of one of the key figures in clinical research: the monitors or clinical research associates (CRAs). Regulatory considerations in safety data collection and further safety studies in post marketing in the form of REMS (risk evaluation and mitigation strategies), has also included a particular emphasis in the entire business enterprise.

> *"...Together with personalized medicine and REMS, two new approaches to clinical development (Adaptive Design and Risk Based Monitoring) have the most... impact on where the jobs are and how would a professional qualify for them..."*

Together with personalized medicine and REMS, two new approaches to clinical development have the most on the impact on where the jobs are and how would a professional qualify for them. They are:

1. Adaptive design
2. Risk based monitoring (RBM)

How these factors in clinical research have impacted the clinical research associate (CRA) jobs?

Lets look at the impact Risk Based Monitoring has in the CRA job description.

This mode of monitoring implies that the sponsor running the studies have access to a very robust IT infrastructure and professionals who will provide for real time or near real time safety and efficacy data collection, and reporting, and monitors would be mostly "centralized" in offices "visualizing" any concern that may prompt an on site monitoring visit, instead of regular periodic visits as it was until recently. This means that the monitor would virtually perform source data verification (patient privacy rules permitting) through access to Electronic Health Records (EHR) and will issue queries without even setting foot at the site. Although some site visits are still going to be necessary, the load will be considerably less.

This mode of monitoring is considered as the next step to streamlining clinical research and containing its costs. I am not going to discuss about RBM here, only it impact on the scope of work of a CRA.

The first thing that many CRAs think is..."there will be much less monitoring jobs out there"... Although a logical conclusion, it does not hold water. First, because we are in a transition period where this kind of monitoring is being implemented, and there will be a lag time until the majority of studies go RBM. Second, there is a limited amount of work hours that one monitor can provide to eSDV (electronically source data verify), issue queries and complete documentation. Nowadays, studies are very large and complicated, and thousands of subjects are enrolled due to the capabilities of handling electronically most of the data. Hence, there will be a need for monitors.

Then the question is what will change in the job description?

We already see the impact of RBM in CRAs job description as follows:

- Remote based CRA
- Virtually based CRA
- In house based CRA
- Centrally based CRA
- Home based CRA

A remote based CRA is a person that will not have an office in the company, nor a little desk when he/she comes (as regional based monitors have when they visit), and all the work will be done utilizing the IT infrastructure that the company provides together with site visits that will be kept at the minimum as required by the protocol. Actually, the employer does not care where you live, as far as you do your job, and meets with the project team regularly.

However, you have to generally live in the country your employer wants you to monitor.

The virtually based CRA, is not so different than the remote based, this is a term mostly utilized in Europe. However, the thing interesting about this position is that the virtual CRA performs all the eSVD off-site and reports electronically. Generally, does not provide for site visits, but prompts which sites have to be monitored in person. I see the implementation of this mode very complicated because of the different patient privacy rules and laws in the EU, and also in other countries that may be involved. Also, the EHR infrastructure has to be fully inter-operable, if hospitals/doctors offices allow external access by third parties located in non secured environments.

The in-house based CRA is a very old mode of activity, however, if RBM is involved, this monitor will perform all the eSVD from the company's office, and reports electronically. Generally, does not provide for site visits, but prompts which sites have to be monitored in person by a regional or remote based monitor.

The centrally based CRA, is a very new as well as old mode of monitoring. Old, because when I joined the industry, more than 25 years ago, before globalization of clinical trials and implementation of good clinical practices, we had all our monitors centrally based, in our head office, and they used to travel all over the country from there. That was a very expensive operation. The "new" centrally based CRA responds to the RBM approach to have the CRA located in a central location where all the IT infrastructure and support will allow the conduct of on line monitoring with access to EHR for eSDV. Although similar to in house based, the name centrally based imply that the monitoring can be centralized by a third-party provider as a CRO (contract research organization) for RBM purposes.

Lastly, the home-based CRA, is the monitor that generally serves a region, and works from his/her home. This monitoring approach has been implemented two decades ago with the aim at reducing travel costs and cost associated with having office space for CRAs that are always on the move.

Therefore, the answer to the above question of what will change in the CRA job description is:

- your physical location, where you are going to work effectively , and
- the approach to monitoring, as to depend heavily on IT infrastructure and support to perform the duties and to a pre-established set of rules that will prompt physical visits to sites

Adaptive design as a factor affecting the monitoring job.

...The adaptive design will provoke that project planning and assignment of monitoring visits will constantly vary...

The type of design of a study will definitively influence how we monitor the study. The adaptive design will provoke that project planning and assignment of monitoring visits will constantly vary according to the interim analysis result and the number of arms or doses that will be dropped. This type of design tend to be a moving target for a project manager as to how to foresee the workload necessary and the budget of a study. Monitors who are involved in clinical trials based on adaptive design, will have to invest lots of resources, previously pre-established in the project plan, to adapt themselves, in a last-minute fashion to changes in the protocol. The last, prompting a cascade of events that the monitor must handle properly to avoid non-compliance. Therefore, I see an increase on the workload of monitors or CRAs who are responsible of studies based on adaptive designs.

> *...I see an increase on the workload of monitors or CRAs who are responsible of studies based on adaptive designs...*

So, where are the CRA Jobs?

They are here and growing!

The opportunities

Your opportunities will shift to a new direction, where you have to add to your set of qualifications, more experience handling electronic systems (EHR, eSource, eCRFs, ePROs, etc).

Also your work will be virtualized in part due to access to new IT infrastructure, travel will be reduced as well as the number of site visits.

Central (virtual) monitoring will greatly increase, creating a large number of in-house or central jobs.

The number of positions available in the near future will depend heavily on,

- regulatory constraints of physical visits,
- access to EHR,
- differences on patient privacy laws in different regions, provision of access to those EHR by hospitals,
- interoperability of electronic systems to allow access, and
- new clinical trial regulations to come (EU 2017)

> *...all CRAs should start adapting to the new trends in the industry and start training and educating themselves on the things to come...*

In summary, all CRAs should start adapting to the new trends in the industry and start training and educating themselves on the things to come.

Originally published on January 20, 2016

In Davos (2016) it was said that 5 million jobs will be lost by 2020, will it include clinical research?

As the World Economic Forum in Davos took place (2016), Alex Gray wrote that ..."Rapid advancements in the fields of technology, such as artificial intelligence and machine learning, and in how we create things, such as robotics, nanotechnology, 3D printing and biotechnology, will dramatically change the characteristics of the global workforce". He pointed out that... "The Fourth Industrial Revolution is changing the workplace fast, and we will need to adapt"..." a Fourth Industrial Revolution is building on the Third, and it is characterized by a fusion of technologies that is blurring the lines between the physical, digital, and biological spheres"....

> ..."*Fourth Industrial Revolution is a fusion of technologies that is blurring the lines between the physical, digital, and biological spheres*"....

That fourth industrial revolution will greatly affect, as is affecting already, the way we develop new therapeutic products. We are already experiencing the enormous impact information technology is having in the way we gather, analyze and report clinical trial data, as well as the power we acquire in performing meta-analysis of data to produce new knowledge. Our clinical research professionals will come from other backgrounds and the once considered soft skills, will constitute and important part of the background, education and knowledge of a clinical research professional: information technology.

I recently published a post about "Where are the clinical research jobs?". There, I discussed briefly that new technologies (IT) and advances in data collection and handling as well as the new approaches to clinical development (Adaptive Design and Risk Based Monitoring), facilitated by IT, will change the scope of work and job descriptions of one of the key figures in clinical research: the monitors or clinical research associates. That change of job description will come together with a redefinition of duties as is source data verification (SDV), safety surveillance or pharmacovigilance, and even patient enrollment. The activities and responsibilities will continue, however the way we perform those will dramatically change.

Yes, the clinical research professional duties will be impacted by the great advances blurring the lines between the physical job (travel and site monitoring), digital (eSDV, ePRO, EHR), and biological spheres (the way we administer treatment).

Yes, the clinical research professional duties will be impacted by the great advances blurring the lines between the physical job (travel and site monitoring), digital (eSDV, ePRO, EHR), and biological spheres (the way we administer treatment).

The other important thing that Alex Gray discuss in his publication is "...According to the Forum's Future of Jobs report, some jobs will be wiped out, others will be in high demand, but all in all, around 5 million jobs will be lost"...

My opinion is that new jobs in clinical research will be created with completely new titles and job descriptions, while others will be disappearing. The new positions that I envision are:

- The Clinical Research Data Scientist (as Alex well introduces the data scientist as a novel and sought after position), (a fusion between a CRA and an IT scientist)
- the Clinical IT auditor, (a fusion between an GCP inspector and an IT auditor)
- Clinical Trial Project Analyst, (a fusion between a CRA or project manager and an IT programmer)
- IT Trial Coordinator (a fusion between a clinical research coordinator and an IT professional)
- IT Regulatory Compliance Associate (fusion between a regulatory associate and IT specialist who will administer all electronic regulatory submissions)
- The Clinical Research Interoperability "guru" (these are going to be almost geniuses who will make sure that the sponsors, CROs and investigators sites IT infrastructure can talk and exchange data, something that now is a challenge)

Wow, I got really creative! However, that is the reality. All our jobs in clinical research will change in shape and form. According to the Future Jobs Report of the World Economic Forum of 2016, 35% of our core skills will change between 2015 and 2020. We will have to adapt and reinvent ourselves to be employable in a new decade that is going to be amassed by our children, born and breed with IT in their lives.

Within the 10 top skills that will impact on employability, Emotional Intelligence and Cognitive Flexibility made it up, while people management and quality control were dropped to lower level of priority. Complex Problem Solving kept the first place, while critical thinking and creativity now follows. I consider that quality control is embedded in our new systems for conducting drug development as part of its nature, without being of less importance but less of a new. What it seems interesting is that people skills is taking a back seat, while critical thinking and creativity are leading. All these points at a reduction in factual human interaction in the future job setting, where individuals will work alone, with virtual interactions that are pre-established by electronic tools where little face to face communication is going to be fostered (I mean real, not virtual). The virtuality of the future jobs will put pressure on the human psyche in such extent that strong Emotional Intelligence and Cognitive Flexibility to jump from the virtual to the real world will be needed to maintain sanity. Here, I can see that new branches in psychology and psychopathology will be created with new specialists who will train and educate on cognitive flexibility.

With this post, I just wanted to share with you my vision and opinion on where the jobs are and are going to be in our field and how to constantly adapt (cognitive flexibility) to be considered a great candidate for a job that is to come.

Originally published on January 21, 2016

Should clinical research in academia comply with a different set of standards to be viable?

Several years ago, and article published in CMAJ(1) bought up the issue of whether we are keeping research participants safe enough? and the burden regulatory requirements, created with the pharmaceutical industry in mind, hinders the ability of doctors of running their own clinical trials. Although, the regulatory burden did not change, actually increased, how are we going to ensure that we are keeping every subject safety up to the same standard (including healthy volunteers).

My opinion has not changed since I posted the following comment:

Clinical Research, keeping the Status Quo or defining the Quo Vadis?

Clinical Research and therapeutic product development has become a very cumbersome experience worldwide, achieving Kafka's delusional proportions. It is understandable the frustration of medical doctors when they embark in the grand endeavor of running clinical trials. I share that for the last 20 years in the industry. We already achieved the mark of 2 billion dollars of development cost per new therapeutic product that reaches the market. That cost is mainly due to.... stringent regulatory requirements. Originally, regulatory requirements for clinical trials were established taking into account the scenario of a pharmaceutical company developing a potential therapeutic product with the intention to apply for a market authorization (NDA/FDA or NDS/Canada). However, subjects- volunteers for clinical trials should have the same rights and protections regardless whether they participate in an industry or academic sponsored clinical trial. This is based on the principles of the Declaration of Helsinki, where the investigator must follow the ethical considerations established, which implies an ethics board review and compliance to local regulations. Nowadays, most of the pharmaceutical sponsored clinical research is global, having international guidelines as Good Clinical Practices as a standard for clinical trials. This document only contains 63 pages, however, we should read the complete title: Guidance for Industry - E6 Good Clinical Practice: Consolidated Guidance (1996). Again, we go back to the original statement that this was definitely developed for the industry.

Now, how come medical doctors that wish to sponsor clinical trials happen to fall in the same category as the industry? , simple, the rationale is that clinical research in human subjects must follow the same rigorous criteria regardless of who the sponsor is, or regardless whether the sponsor wishes or not to apply for a market authorization.

The introduction of these international standards did impact the industry as a whole and the cost of development only skyrocketed. The main source of incremental cost is indeed quality control (monitoring) and quality assurance (standards operational procedures and auditing). However, how far we can go in assuring quality of data and ensuring patient protection? Note that the regulation establishes that the sponsor must ensure adequate monitoring, that is commensurable to risk. However, the issue is how much is adequate?

The other point that (you) make is that the clinical trials that academic sponsors (medical doctors as sponsors) run are with lower risks. I do not agree that clinical trials run by the academia are of lower risk even though a marketed product is utilized. The risk inherent to utilizing a marketed drug in a new indication, not approved, therefore of unknown safety, is not because of the pharmacokinetics or adverse events profile, but because of possible lack of efficacy, or use in a different dose range or dosage, or even in a patient population not approved in the product labeling.

I do agree that the drug or therapeutic product development process is not sustainable, and a change is needed to allow the required research to advance in human therapeutics. I also understand that there is limited expertise in ethics board members to assess ongoing safety of clinical studies or the complex protocol designs, not to mention the review timeliness that are longer and longer. However, I also consider that medical doctors acting as principal investigators and sponsors should be properly trained in drug development process and regulatory requirements to properly conduct clinical research. It is important to highlight that clinical research is not medical practice.

Also, I do not consider that the academia should have different standards than the industry for clinical research on human subjects, I believe that the entire therapeutic product development process should and must be modernized to allow faster proof of concept, better initial evaluation, and streamlined regulatory process. The billion-dollar question is how to achieve that without compromising the subjects' right and welfare and data quality.

The answer may rely on resolving first the dichotomies between business or science, commercial product or human health and profits or human value.

The proposal to revamp the regulatory process of drug development can only be laudable, and I believe that we in Canada can set a new standard of clinical research and achieve the same degree of confidence and international recognition with New Good Clinical Practices – a guideline for all sponsors, investigators and ethics review boards.

Having written this response 6 years ago, begs the question, what did change in the regulatory sphere to increase subject safety and streamline the process? not too much...

Originally published on January 24, 2016

(1)   CMAJ ,July 13, 2010 182:E428

Is your Nursing Job Burning You Out? Have you Though about Clinical Research?

For many years, I have been approached by nurses all over the world, while either working on sites doing GCP inspections, training and conducting seminars or selecting investigators, with a very common question: do you think I qualify for a job in clinical research?

My answer was very simple: YES!, and then I followed it with my own question, why?

The majority of nurses that inquired whether they qualify for a job in clinical research stated that burnout, long hours, together with a growing family as the main reasons to look for a job outside from direct patient care.

Most of the nurses I talked to did not have a general idea of what a clinical research job entitled and how they can make the transition. That is why I decided to write this post, so professional nurses do not have to wonder which path to follow.

The path to a clinical research job

As a nurse, you have a very sound educational and patient related experience that is highly regarded in clinical research. However, it is not enough. Depending on the type of job you select as your path from direct patient care to clinical research, you will have to train in rules and regulations, as well as good clinical practices, and the drug development process. Training and education may not be exactly what a person who wants a career change has in mind. However, clinical research is a highly regulated business enterprise, and you have to be very much knowledgeable of regulatory requirements and the clinical research process to increase your chances of being offered a job. Very seldom and employer will hire you without those qualifications.

The majority of nurses also told me that they cannot put time aside to go back to school. So, the most doable option is to train on line. There are online training programs organized by colleges and notable universities, however those programs are not necessarily available anytime and anywhere, however they are a very good option. Having in mind accessibility to training, and wanting to make professional resources available for our investigators and clients, we came to the idea to offer training through an eLearning platform that allows nurses and other health professionals train on their own time, anytime and anywhere, even using their smartphones and tablets. Nevertheless, my advice is ..."do your own research as of what programs suits you best"... (click here if you want to start working on your path).

What job a professional nurse can do in clinical research?

There are many jobs/positions a nurse can qualify in clinical research and be very productive. The following three are the ones that nurses are most successful as the entry point in clinical research.

The Clinical Research Coordinator. This job title applies to science professionals who assist the clinical trial investigator (principal investigator) on running the clinical trial at the investigators site. This is a great entry point, most of the positions are within hospital settings, so nurses already know the environment. The pro is that the hours are regular, and there is no travel involved. The stress level is not as high as when you are tending to patients in providing health care, since clinical research is not medical practice, is research. Nevertheless, it is provided within a healthcare setting and may be provided in conjunction with health care. Being a certified nurse makes you, as a coordinator, able to provide for services you are qualified for, and therefore have the advantage above other professionals in the very same job. As I always say.."the nurse coordinator is the administrative arm of the principal investigator..."

The Clinical Research Coordinators Assistant. This is a more junior job compared to the above. Mainly you would assist the coordinator in the required tasks to run smoothly a clinical trial at a site.

The Clinical Research Associate (CRA).

These jobs are within a pharmaceutical company or a contract research organization. It requires travel, depending on the type of CRA, can go from 25% (seldom) to more than 75% of the time (in most of the cases). These are very well-paid jobs, and experience is a must.

What are the advantages and disadvantages of a nursing vs. clinical research job?

This is a question that always follows after we start the discussion. I consider that there are lots of advantages, and only a few comparative disadvantages.

Let's look at the advantages:

- Regular business hours (seldom work on weekends or evenings, only if required by the study protocol)
- Health care setting, what gives familiar environment
- Direct interaction with people
- Real possibilities for advancement in the industry
- Be part of new therapeutic approaches
- Very limited travel (may be only for training)
- Interaction with industry professionals at a scientific level
- Less stress (as compared to a nurse job)
- May work from home (home based CRA)
- May work part time in certain places

The few disadvantages I may see,

- Fixed income (unless working as a contractor)
- Work on weekdays during business work hours (I consider that an advantage)
- More administrative work
- High level of documentation handling
- Salaries may differ compared to a specialized nurse

Originally Published on January 26, 2016

Patient Centered Medicine vs. Patient Centric Medicine and vs. Personalized Medicine

In Clinical Research as in Medical Practice, there has been a flurry of misconceptions and misunderstanding of the concepts of Patient Centric Medicine, Patient Centered Medicine and Personalized Medicine. Some professionals use the terms interchangeably yielding to further puzzling in patients and others. Let me bring some light to the concepts, so everyone can be in the same page in the conversation.

Where do all these new concepts came from?

First, let's see why these concepts have been developed. Here I have some insights:

The main issue was how to implement new revolutionizing technologies to improve the way medical care is delivered efficiently.

Also, to give an insight to patients that they are going to be greatly benefited by new technologies and approaches to their care.

Lastly, to create a frame of work for scientists and governments in function of where the funds are going to go to achieve the first.

Basically, we needed to reinvent medicine and delivery of care to include those new technologies as key for great improvement.

What is Patient Centered Medicine?

Going back in the history of the term, the Committee on Quality of Health Care in America, IOM, published a document titled " Crossing the Quality Chasm" A New Health Care system for the 21st. Century"(2001). This document coined the concept Patient-Centered Care as "providing care that is respectful of and responsive to individual patient preferences, needs, and values and ensuring that patient values guide all clinical decisions".

***Patient Centered Care ...** " providing care that is respectful of and responsive to individual patient preferences, needs, and values and ensuring that patient values guide all clinical decisions".*

Further, the NIH elaborated the term as "health care that establishes a partnership among practitioners, patients, and their families (when appropriate) to ensure that decisions respect patients' wants, needs and preferences and solicit patients' input on the education and support they need to make decisions and participate in their own care".

Basically, patient-centered medicine (care) involves the patient (and their families) in the decision of how care is delivered meanwhile key for that decision is to provide with accurate information and support.

What is Patient Centric Medicine?

Patient centric medicine is based on the fact that the patient is the source of the information and point of interaction for the delivery of care. This centricity is possible due to new technologies that allow patients to produce their own data easily and submit it directly to the health provider to guide the medical care decisions. In clinical research, that concept has been the key in data collection though electronic patient reported outcome systems (ePRO), to allow the ongoing collection of safety and efficacy data to proactively make near real time decisions on the subjects' participation.

Patient centric medicine is based on the fact that the patient is the source of the information and point of interaction for the delivery of care.

It is important to know that the concept is unintentionally interchanged with patient centered medicine, especially when looking into Affordable Care Act and its interpretations.

What is Personalized Medicine?

__Personalized medicine.__(is) "the use of genomic, epigenomic, exposure and other data to define individual patterns of disease, potentially leading to better individual treatment"

Although the concept is not new, National Academy of Sciences (NAS) defines personalized medicine as "the use of genomic, epigenomic, exposure and other data to define individual patterns of disease, potentially leading to better individual treatment." It is used interchangeably as "precision medicine," "stratified medicine," "targeted medicine," and "pharmacogenomics," I personally like the concept of pharmacogenomics, whereas the analysis and identification of specific genomic markers would allow pinpoint the right medicine where the patient will respond and not have serious adverse events.

As you can see, they are three completely different concepts, that once well defined and understood, will allow its implementation to health care in a seamless manner.

Originally published on January 27, 2016

Depression treatment tools emerging as patient centric medicine is implemented

The overall response rate to depression drug treatment is less than 50%, with lower than 30% of patients achieving remission with initial drug therapy (1). This leaves patients exposed to trial and error coping with the burden of disease for months without improvement and dropping out of treatment because lack of efficacy. Some depressive episodes resolve by themselves (?) when the external factor is eliminated. Depression as a condition, if not treated either with psychological intervention or drug therapy, becomes of a great impact on the patient's life, family and the society at large. In my opinion, depression together with anxiety disorders are amongst the most prevalent conditions in our societies, leaving primary health care providers to take action to improve the heath of their patients.

Depression, as well as other psychiatric conditions, are very hard to objectively diagnose since there is no lab test or diagnostic imaging tool to see the disease, measure it and determine its therapy. Mostly, depression is intuitively treated at the level of primary care, what makes it a further challenge.

The lack of objective diagnostic tools together with having most of the antidepressant treatments prescribed at primary care level, makes depression, a pervasive health issue.

A recent advance published online on January 20, 2016 in the Lancet Psychiatry provides with a new tool based on depression diagnosed patient-reported data (here is the patient centric aspect) where they were able to identify 25 variables that were most predictive of treatment outcome. The group applied the data to train a computer-learning algorithm to predict clinical remission with citalopram. The model, which was internally cross-validated, predicted outcomes with accuracy "significantly above chance" (64.6%, $P < .0001$), to identify a responder to first treatment with citalopram. This kind of new tools increase the probability for a qualified health care provider to precisely prescribe an antidepressant and have a higher chance of yielding remission without trial and error.

As you can see I utilize the term "qualified health care provider" very carefully to stress the need to focus prescription of antidepressants at the level of psychiatry and not as a primary health care intervention. Otherwise, we should greatly strengthen the qualifications of primary health care providers to be able to implement a validated diagnostic and prescription protocol. This new tool is a step towards that, however we must proceed with care.

New approaches to treatment involve CBT (cognitive behavioral therapy) with or without drug treatment, increase the success of treatment considerably. Access is the other variable in the outcome of treatment.

Nevertheless, first, how can we effectively diagnose to streamline treatment? how to predict precisely the outcome? how to determine if a patient is going to respond to treatment avoiding 6 to 8 weeks of trial and error per drug? how to ensure that qualified doctors prescribe and follow-up on treatment in the long term?

Originally Published on January 29, 2016

About Pregnancy and Clinical Trials, Really?

A recently published article (JAMA. 2018;320(20):2077-2078. doi:10.1001/jama.2018.17716), discusses the challenge of having pregnant women as patient volunteers in clinical research. Their hypothesis is that … "Preventing pregnant women from participating in clinical trials is well intentioned but misguided…". Further, they elaborate that the biggest challenge is that …" For ethical committee approval, study interventions in pregnancy must directly benefit or pose minimal risk to the mother and fetus, and often consent must be obtained from both parents…". For which the article concludes that …" Thus, more than 80% of pregnant patients are routinely prescribed therapies that have not been studied in pregnancy. Given the limited amount of safety data, it is largely unknown if medications could harm patients, which interventions are truly effective, or whether it is safe to delay treatment until after pregnancy…". This sentence establishes clearly that the safety of the pregnant woman, and not the fetus, is considered in the hypothesis, making fetal safety not a matter of issue.

It is important to note that the authors acknowledge that the FDA enacted policies to provide special protections to pregnant women in the 1960's and 1970's due to …" unanticipated complications from in utero exposure …" to thalidomide and diethylstillbestrol downplaying completely the terrible deformities and suffering that children born from mothers taking those drugs still endure.

Nonetheless, the article makes a case for having pregnant women participate regularly in clinical research regardless of direct benefit due to pregnancy or to fetus as they expand that …" Developing clear, actionable guidelines to include pregnant women in trials could contribute essential knowledge to the understanding of disease and its treatment…"

The authors of this article, in my opinion, provide a prejudiced approach to pregnancy as a human state, in which no special protections should be provided and that a pregnant woman does not necessitate further shield from potentially noxious substances, implying that the developing fetus is not a matter of concern but represented as a potential unanticipated complication. They further establish a completely inaccurate inference in which they consider that pregnant women were put in the category of special populations because they are at the same level of need for protections because they are unable to decide for themselves and pairing them to children or mentally challenged subjects. That comes from their position that "…Pregnant women are fully able to weigh the ethical implications of health decisions they make for themselves and their fetuses, especially when given adequate counseling about their conditions and treatment options…"

It is very worrisome to read that pregnancy is believed, by some, a mental handicap. I consider that pregnant women were and are always able to make health decisions by themselves and that with proper education and information, proceed with their own care in a safe, ethical and principled manner. Otherwise, humanity will not be here now.

All the examples of pregnant women in clinical research presented in the mentioned article are evidence as of why more pregnant women are needed in clinical trials, directly impact their own health or to treat/prevent potential fetal disease. Therefore, they are in concurrence with the existent requirements for protections of pregnant women in clinical research.

It is very important to understand that for the benefit of the subject, fetus and the society at large, strict barriers and very thorough ethics review and consenting process of the pregnant women in clinical trials with relevant inclusion of the father, are key to guarantee the safety of the mother and the fetus.

Let's elaborate on the thinking presented in the mentioned article regarding the barriers to include pregnant women in clinical trials.

Barrier #1:…" the designation of pregnant women as "vulnerable"..

The article considers that women are not vulnerable and should not considered as such because …" these women make ongoing medical decisions for themselves and their fetuses when faced with limited safety evidence"…

I consider that the article is misguided in their opinion that vulnerability is correlated to the mental ability to make decisions. To make an opinion, we must refer to the proper definition of the word vulnerability that is "the quality or state of being exposed to the possibility of being attacked or harmed…". Therefore, the state of vulnerability of a pregnant woman comes from the fact that there is a potential for exposure to a noxious or unknown substance (considered here as exposure to harm) with unknown consequences for her or her unborn child. Vulnerability does not come from the fact of inability to make a decision because of her state.

The article further proposed that pregnant women be defined as "scientifically complex"…and that … "pregnancy does not alter a woman's capacity for autonomous decision making". Again, the article erroneously understands vulnerability as diminished capacity and lack of autonomy, being those two completely different concepts and thus not interchangeable.

Barrier #2:..." federal regulations do not define "acceptable risk" to a woman or fetus"...

In their discussion, the article refers to the Common Rule, that is very well established and properly assigned, in which ..." if trial participation will not directly benefit the [pregnant]woman or fetus, risk must not be greater than minimal..." as participating in daily life.

The article ponders that ..." how a woman or family defines reasonable risk may differ depending on their view of the anticipated opportunities and expectations for the pregnancy and future baby, as well as the urgency of the clinical question...". First and foremost, risk for trial participation is not defined or calculated by the participating subject. The subject can only agree or not to assume the risk proposed in the informed consent form for their participation in the clinical trial. It is my opinion that the article seems to understand that reasonable risk is a fluid concept that varies depending on the situation, as are opportunities, expectations and urgency of the clinical question.

Actually, the regulations establish that reasonable risks are assessed by ethics boards when a protocol is submitted for review, in which, considering rules and regulations, make a decision (either positive, negative or asking more questions) on clinical trials. Further ethics boards, must consider additional safeguards for vulnerable populations, including pregnant woman because of potential harm to them and/or the unborn child, and not because diminished capacity. As such, risk is not a fluid concept, and the volunteer subject is not qualified to make the decision on the level of risk, but either participate or not in the trial. Otherwise, why do we have ethics boards and investigators with express responsibilities towards special populations? Additionally, risk cannot be defined as high, medium or low. Risk should be evaluated based on concrete evidence and properly assessed in function of the requirements of the law.

Barrier #3: ..." A third barrier is the perceived legal risk if the fetus or mother has an adverse outcome."

The article considers that the third barrier is the legal/financial assumption of the responsibilities for unanticipated complications due to failed risk assessment or inclusion of subjects that do not qualify for a clinical trial in experimentation. To consider limiting the responsibilities of sponsors and/or investigators for serious "unexpected" adverse events when they decide to include pregnant subjects in clinical trials, is to diminish the robustness of the clinical trial process, opening doors to irresponsible research. Having strict systems into place to safeguard trial subjects, deters unscrupulous research. Unfortunately, legal systems put into place to safeguard patients at large are abused for monetary gain, and that is not part of this discussion, but cannot be used as evidence to diminish safeguards in the future.

It is important to note that the "Report to the Secretary, Health and Human Services, Congress, TASK FORCE ON RESEARCH SPECIFIC TO PREGNANT WOMEN AND LACTATING WOMEN" issued recommendations in September 2018 titled "Task Force on Research Specific to Pregnant Women and Lactating Women Recommendations" that derive from the issue that pregnant women and lactating women are often excluded from clinical research that could ultimately help these populations. The task force issued 15 recommendations in which they highlight that ..." the[re is] need to alter cultural assumptions that have significantly limited scientific knowledge of therapeutic product safety, effectiveness, and dosing for pregnant and lactating women. The cultural shift is necessary to emphasize the importance and public health significance of building a knowledge base to inform medical decision-making for these populations."

That refers to the cultural assumption (that have significantly limited scientific knowledge) to the evidence provided in the 1960's and 1970's of catastrophic adverse events to drugs (e.g. Thalidomide) in pregnant women that produced children with severe handicaps. Those children in the photographs are real evidence and not a cultural assumption and should not be downplayed or ignored. Those children are now adults who bear the consequences of lax regulations of the time that allowed pregnant women use those drugs without previous clinical safety data. Having extensive worldwide clinical evidence, regulators rightly limited, but never excluded, the participation of pregnant women in studies where there is an unknown risk to the fetus.

Having said that, in the aim to obtain objective evidence of safety and efficacy of treatments that directly benefit pregnant women and/or the fetus, it is very important that any research is conducted in the context of all the provisions already available for their safeguard. Further, preclinical studies provide limited evidence, and the pharmacology in healthy volunteers support human safety in general. Pharmacological properties of drugs provide direct evidence of potential excretion in human milk, however their effect in breastfeeding children may not be inferred.

The regulations, as presently established, do not curb vaccine studies or any other drug study that directly benefit pregnant women and the fetus. However, they establish special provisions for the safety and well being of the population that cannot be diminished for the sake of streamline research. For example, the flu vaccine is specifically recommended in pregnant women. Millions of pregnant women were exposed to those vaccines to date, and robust evidence to support the use on the population exists. Therefore, exposure data should be collected from REGISTRIES of pregnant women taking medications, that are not subject to regulatory constraints of clinical trials, and that still can provide valuable data for prescribing and dosing decisions without purposely exposing pregnant women and their fetuses to unknown risks for the sake of informing medical decision. Those registries collect worldwide data, providing valuable information on the safety of therapeutic products.

Conditions that drugs intend to treat during pregnancy, that are not related to pregnancy, are mostly well known, and data on safety of drugs to treat those diseases during pregnancy is available (e.g. antiepileptic drugs). Pregnancy should be considered when a woman has an underlying condition that requires extensive treatments and avoided in most of the cases. Therefore, proper education and information should be available.

The potential of severe injury due to exposing pregnant women to drugs (catastrophic adverse event) is exponentially increased since there is a potential for injury to the mother, to the fetus or both. Since the experimentation can affect a new generation, producing comparable effects already observed in the past with e.g. thalidomide, extreme precaution and commensurate compensation for injury are not a matter of barrier to be eliminated for the sake of disease understanding.

Additionally, in the US, there are further health insurance implications to the mother and the child who participate(d) in clinical trials during pregnancy. For example, most health insurance companies deny care for clinical research injuries, and that becomes responsibility of the sponsor. Also, future access to health care for the baby born from a mother who participated in a clinical trial, where the investigational drug might have produced "unintended complications", can be subject to claw backs or deem ineligible.

In conclusion:

- Clinical research to determine safety and efficacy of a study drug in pregnant women is regulated and not excluded.
- Safeguards are in place to guarantee that vulnerable subjects (in this case pregnant women) are not exposed to unnecessary risks to her and her developing fetus, and ethics boards are the decision makers for risk assessment.
- Safety data on certain drugs used during pregnancy is known.
- Limiting liability for adverse events in pregnant women during clinical trials, only diminishes the safeguards in place to protect subjects in clinical research
- Reducing barriers for clinical research in pregnant women may expose, unnecessarily, fetuses to unknown risks otherwise they will not be exposed to, for the sake to contribute essential knowledge to the understanding of disease and its treatment. A proper assessment of risk benefits should be included.

Originally Published on December 3, 2018

5 Common Misconceptions for the cause of the Health Care Crisis

Walking through hospital hallways and doctors' offices all around the globe, while working in clinical research, made me rationalize about the different approaches in delivering health care. Hence, there are many misconceptions that I consider should be addressed to find a doable solution to the health care crisis.

Misconception #1 – *Health Care Costs are only going to increase*

If we consider that health care costs are directly proportional to the population size and age, then the hypothesis is correct, however, it is not. We assume that the more the people, the higher the cost, and that is very far from the truth. Here is why:

We cannot accept to the status quo regarding health care. Population health improves with access to education, clean water, healthy food and appropriate housing. Also, health should improve with preventative measures that in turn will reduce ER and doctor visits.

Misconception #2 – *Preventative Medicine is doing well*

Preventative medicine has not been exploited or implemented into the context of health care in a manner to produce a real impact in population health. Vaccination is not the only preventative tool, and actually over vaccination may be a curse more than a solution. Nevertheless, vaccination has been a turning point in health and prevention. However, other diseases have replaced infectious diseases. The majority of cardiovascular diseases, diabetes, hypertension and even cancer, can be prevented or even reversed with effective education in healthy eating and weight control. Health care systems should implement rewards to people who keep a healthy weight, do not smoke, drink alcohol or use recreational drugs. Conversely, premiums should be applied when people are overweight, consume alcohol, recreational drugs or smoke. Running effective educational campaigns and using social media to impact youth, will reduce health care needs in the short and long term.

Misconception #3- *ER visits will only take longer*

Actually, the triage system in hospitals globally is completely different, and the impact on care is seen very evidently. In Canada and the UK the length of ER visits as well as lack of hospital beds has become of critical proportions. The reason is very simple, patient management from the moment the show-up at ER lacks of proper triage, where all patients are treated as emergency cases instead of being properly re-routed. A solution should include a health care provider, preferably a doctor, greeting the patient at the door and deciding if it is an emergency or not with a few questions, and provide for care on the spot or advise and educate the patient about his/her options of health care in the future. People should be given more education on how the system works and doctors should instruct patients on who should they contact if they are not available instead of sending them to the ER. We go back to the hypothesis that education is the best way to prevent disease and reduce health care costs.

Just let me tell you an anecdotal story. I was at the ER in an eastern European country, and although there were lots of people, all of them were greeted at the door and triaged immediately to get the best care available. While looking how do they work, I saw a young doctor greeting an elderly man who was walking oddly and said..."hi grandpa, did you fall off your chair? Or tripped in the rug?, and the old man answered..."oh child, I did indeed fell from my chair..." the next I heard was..."nurse ...wheelchair...straight to x-rays...here is the order... someone will be with you to take your info while in x-ray room"... All the conversation lasted 30 seconds. The old man was seen, x-rayed, treated and discharged in less than 30 minutes.

Another anecdote was when I was in Argentina, where a patient had severe heart failure, and was developing pulmonary edema. The ambulance arrived in less than 10 minutes from the moment the call was placed, and there was a doctor in the ambulance. The doctor provided emergency care before she was taken to the ambulance in such a manner that she was being already stabilized. It took 10 minutes to get to the hospital, where they were already waiting for her. She was immediately sent to cardiovascular ICU, and all the tests were proceeding, the only wait time was to receive the test results that came in 30 minutes, although treatment was initiated. From the moment the call was placed to the time she started her treatment, it only passed less than 20 minutes. Tests were only to verify the diagnosis. She was discharged in 3 days.

Misconception #4 – *People will be taking more medication in the future*

This misconception ties with the first one, where health care costs are only going to increase with population. The truth of the matter is that people are taking twice more drugs that in the past, and it is believed that they are really necessary. This is very far from the truth. The only reason people are taking more medications is because they are prescribed more, and that disease prevention is considered to be with more medications. For instance, cardiovascular diseases and diabetes are not tackled with real education, diet and weight control, but with anti-hypertensives, cholesterol lowering drugs and/or sugar lowering drugs. Hence this hypothesis is tied with misconception #2.

Misconception #5 – *Cheaper drugs is the solution to lowering health care costs*

Drugs comprise about 15 % of the total health care cost. Having cheaper drugs will not impact on health care costs in a significant manner, especially if the number of prescriptions increase. Again, preventing diseases that are related to lifestyle are the best bet in reducing health care costs. Then, drugs will only be used when are really necessary steering R&D to unmet needs with real ROI.

Therefore, we wrongly believe that health care costs are only going to increase, preventative medicine is doing well, ER visits will only take longer, people will be taking more medication in the future, and cheaper drugs is the solution to lowering health care costs. Therefore, health care policies are being steered towards addressing those hypotheses with more investment in hospital beds, medications and access to care at different levels foreseeing an increase in cardiovascular diseases and diabetes, without addressing the underlying problem of lack of education, access to healthy foods and creating healthy lifestyles that could be rewarded with financial incentives.

It is time to give preventative medicine the front seat and create an environment where people will have access to information and knowledge to maintain and improve their health. At the end of the day, we all want to be healthy…

It is time to give preventative medicine the front seat and create an environment where people will have access to information and knowledge to maintain and improve their health. At the end of the day, we all want to be healthy...

I am not a health care administrator nor have any direct involvement in delivering service. I am a clinical scientist trained mainly in observation, data collection, analysis and reporting.

Originally published on March 20, 2018

Opioid overdose due to dose dumping....

In the quest to deter the illegal use of regulatory approved opioid prescription drugs, slow release/tamper resistant delivery forms came into the market with the promise to effectively reduce the misuse of the drug. The World Health Organization (WHO) published recently that about 15 million people suffer from opioid dependence, and that also an estimated 69 000 people die from opioid overdose each year worldwide. Whereas the CDC published that only during 2014, a total of 47,055 drug deaths occurred due to opioid OD in the United States. In general, a 200% increase in the rate of overdose deaths involving opioids was registered in the last decade. Overall, the US bears the brunt of abuse, overdose and deaths due to the liberal prescription influenced by the presumed safety of newly developed dosage forms.

Let's examine the new approaches to deliver solid oral forms that can increase the safety concerns and why.

In theory, slow /timed /extended release forms are created in such manner that a full day (or a longer period) dosage of drug is available in one pill that a patient is to take daily or periodically as per their doctor's instructions. They are very convenient and increase compliance.

These solid forms are manufactured with the purpose of providing a single pill that must not be divided, or sliced, in any way. It is very important that the patient takes the whole pill as it is provided by the manufacturer, since an entire days' worth of dose may be in there, if not more. If the pill's integrity is damaged in any way, shape, or form, it may produce what is called dose dumping, and therefore you may end up having one entire day's worth of medication released inside your body all at once, instead of it being slowly delivered to you in the course of the day. That may produce serious toxic effects, even catastrophic/lethal ones, depending on the type of the drug the pill contained.

These slow/extended/timed release forms are generally manufactured either with a mesh on the pill that dissolves slowly inside your digestive tract, making the drug slowly available during the day, or they are compressed into layers with different solubility patterns, or there might be some other type of release mechanism that will allow you to take the minimum number of pills in a day.

The safety of these delivery forms depends on the integrity and quality of the pill. Be very careful when handling them, and make sure that you follow your health care provider's instructions.

Misuse of the slow/extended release form, breaking, grinding, snorting, injecting etc. are all NOT INTENDED uses, and therefore constitutes a serious safety concern. In all cases, dose dumping occurs, and the subject ends up in ER or worse.

Good Clinical Practices (GCP/ICH) R2 Integrated Addendum has changed the Clinical Trials landscape, have you noticed?

In November 2016, the Integrated Addendum to ICH E6 (R1) : 'Guideline for Good Clinical Practice has been issued'. Have you noticed the changes and how are they going to impact your clinical trials business enterprise? Actually, I did.

I consider this addendum to be the most profound change on how clinical trials are run.

These substantial changes will have a great impact on monitoring, data management and validation, quality and risk management, as well as extended responsibilities of investigators and sponsors of clinical trials. The financial and logistical impact is going to be felt very soon when an in depth understanding of the requirements is achieved. May be, unintentionally, this revision of the guideline stressed key compliance points that were assumed but not properly implemented in the past. Nevertheless, there will be an implicit cost to implementation, as well as retraining of clinical trial personnel that will be felt across the entire industry.

The question is, how prepared is the industry and other stakeholders to comply with new standards that require a complete revamp on the corporate culture of clinical trials enterprise.

In my opinion, depending on the stakeholder (pharmaceutical company/CRO/third party provider, etc) many of the aspects of the new revision, were implemented or contemplated as nice to have, or do. With time and cost constraints, activities as RCA (root cause analysis) and CAPA (corrective and preventative action) were never performed in a standardized or systematically as in pharmaceutical manufacturing. Even the concept is foreign to most monitors or other clinical trial professionals.

Centralized monitoring seems to be the motto of the monitoring process, relying heavily on electronic and computerized systems to drive patient safety oversight. Routine physical site visits will be phased out for very well planned and documented Monitoring Strategy that will assume safety risks with statistical approach and hence trigger otherwise programmed visits.

Although we have the FDA 21 CFR 11 for Electronic Records and Signatures, for example, qualification and validation of computerized systems was done in an environment oblivious of GCP itself or the clinical trial process/requirements. It was seldom incorporated as an SOP in clinical trials management or as part of exhaustive quality assurance inspections.

Originally published on April 6, 2017

5 big mistakes in Consenting Clinical Trial Subjects have to do with Vulnerability

Provisions for the protection of human subjects have been sanctioned and revised, and in the 60 years after the Nuremberg code, we are still struggling to address the issue of subject vulnerability and the moral and ethical implications of medical experimental procedures.

In my opinion, patients, per se, due to the immanent status of perceived disease, are vulnerable subjects regardless of their apparent condition. Further, when a person becomes a patient, assumes the position of vulnerability seeking help from a professional to mitigate his or her issue. The state of "disease" intrinsically diminishes the person's ability to care for themselves (e.g. if you have a bacterial infection and high fever with chills, you feel weak and vulnerable and go to the doctor to help you with your care).

> "*patients, per se, due to the immanent status of perceived disease, are vulnerable subjects regardless of their apparent condition*"

Vulnerability comes from the fact that a person is no able to retain control of their life situation and or protect themselves against threats to their integrity (physical and mental). That vulnerability varies in degrees and has to do more with the person's perception than factual state.

The state of "disease" intrinsically diminishes the person's ability to care for themselves

It is logical to assume that there are different levels of vulnerability, mainly, a child is vulnerable, just because is a child and is unable to care for him/ herself. A bedridden person is vulnerable because depends on others for their care and sustainability of life. A senile patient cannot understand their situation and become as dependent as a child. These examples are the very evident examples of subject vulnerability for which the special protections exists. However, what about all other persons that perceive their position as vulnerable because they depend on someone else for their health or well-being?

The obvious response to vulnerability is to protect from harm. Even Hippocrates (460-370BC) was aware that the intrinsic vulnerability due to the perceived state of disease exposes patients to harm. Therefore, he established the very well-known concept to medical interventions..."do not do harm" ...

Creating special protections to only established vulnerable subjects, may not address the vulnerability of all other ones that do not fall into that evident category.

Although it may be a very important topic for ethicists, the point of the matter is, that until you are exposed to vulnerability in the health care setting, directly or as a health care professional, it is not possible to understand the great challenge. Therefore, currently established provisions for clinical trial subjects may not provide enough protection as they should, because a lack of understanding of what a vulnerable subject is....until you are exposed to vulnerability in the health care setting, directly or as a health care professional, it is not possible to understand the great challenge.

In the clinical trial setting, there is an effective need to enroll eligible subjects as soon as possible and meet all the criteria for study completion. Clinical trial subjects are required to sign a consent form to enroll. Those consent forms are long, complex, ambiguous, self-limiting on explaining the purpose of the intervention, and at the end too cumbersome for most patients to read, understand and sign. This challenge has reduced considerably the number of people keen on participating, and therefore, pharmaceutical companies had to resort to globalizing studies to meet their enrollment targets. The need to provide evidence of understanding, beyond the signature in the document, made the process more cumbersome, and sometimes subjects just give up and leave, or gave in, and "trust" that everything will be OK.

Below, I am highlighting, in my opinion, the 5 mistakes in preconceptions of clinical trial subjects' vulnerabilities, for which provisions are made through ethics standards and reviews, and the consenting process. Nevertheless, everything goes down to the signing of a consent document by a vulnerable subject, established as a volunteer.

The 5 mistakes in the preconception regarding vulnerability of clinical trial subjects are:

1. **UNDERSTANDING.** Obtaining a signature and, may be, answering to written questions to the procedures described in the consent document are not evidence enough of understanding of the experimental procedure. Vulnerable subjects are prone to give in, and go with the flow, because they want to be relieved of their

suffering, and perceive that participation in the study may do that. There is no need to "influence" the subject, because their intrinsic vulnerability of a perceive state of disease, makes them complaisant.

2.   **FEAR**. Patients do fear of their perceived diseased state. Fear from pain and suffering is intrinsic to human nature. Fear makes the patient more vulnerable. More so if they have a psychiatric condition (e.g. depression) in which limited processing of thought may blur their ability for reasoning.

3.   **EXPECTATIONS**. Patients who are looking to participate in a clinical trial, are actively seeking a solution to their disease state. Clinical trials may, through common thought in the general population, be construed as a viable option to care. (e.g. …"Clinical trials offer hope for many people…"…"participants with an illness or disease also participate … to possibly receive the newest treatment…")

4.   **LANGUAGE AND CULTURE**. Language and cultural behaviours have been a challenge from the beginning of clinical research, in which patients may feel obliged to agree to participate. In that case, they are presented with very well written documents they barely understand, and their cultural setting does not allow them to refuse a doctor's recommendation. The culture always puts a patient in a lesser position where due to the vulnerability of a diseased state, makes them agree to interventions they may not understand.

5.   **VOLUNTARISM**. Participants in clinical trials are all considered volunteers, deciding to participate freely, and in which they do not expect compensation or reward other than the participation itself. The concept of voluntarism is very important, since it can be construed in many ways unless specifically stated. Depending on the line of thought, voluntarism may contrast intellect, and therefore decisions are made based on beliefs rather than knowledge, while on the other hand, it assumes reason.

Assuming that the challenges regarding knowledge, fear, expectations, language & culture and voluntarism are properly addressed, the clinical trial process might unduly expose vulnerable subjects (patients) to experimental interventions without the corresponding protections and scrutiny, provoking unnecessary suffering (through unfulfilled expectations and unanticipated risks).

Taking into account that less than 5% of all the investigated therapeutic products reach the market as viable drugs, subjects that participated in the other more than 95% of the failed products, contributed their time and health to help demonstrate that a particular drug product is not suitable, exposing themselves to the risk of lack of efficacy, no treatment due to placebo, or unforeseen or serious adverse events.

Unless the immanent patients' vulnerabilities are properly addressed, there will continue to be ethical concerns that will only challenge patient protections further.

Originally published on January 16, 2018

The New Frontier in Health Care - Artificial Intelligence, a brief opinion

Part I - Let's work on the concept of AI

In the last few decades, the concept of "artificial intelligence (AI)" has occupied the minds of the brightest and most intelligent people of our planet. It is a new concept, AI was coined in the mid-20th century and was more of science-fiction than reality at the time. However, in the first 18 years of the 21st century we are talking very seriously about AI and its impact on humanity. The important thing that we need to clarify is what AI means, although many AI minds do not think that a definition will impact the final outcome of the technology.

In my opinion, AI is "the performance of a finite task or tasks by a machine, using defined new or established data and processes, in the most efficient manner, to procure the most successful outcome". The success can be measured in cost, efficiency, or quality of deliverable.

AI is " the performance of a finite task or tasks by a machine, using defined new or established data and processes, in the most efficient manner, to procure the most successful outcome".

Now, the challenge in the label "artificial intelligence" comes from the perspective of the neophyte to rationalize the concept "intelligence" as intrinsic to the machine itself without human intervention, and here is where the scientific community failed to explain to the common person of what are they talking about.

Computers or super computers are not intelligent, they are machines that, and when turned off, they are very efficient in accumulating dust. "Artificial intelligence" algorithms and routines are nothing more than human designed. Therefore, the concept of AI is a misconception, since the machines by themselves cannot do anything unless are properly programmed and data is provided to answer a particular question.

At this point I will give myself the liberty to redefine the concept, to make it closer to what it is. I am re-branding "artificial intelligence" to "Human Enhanced Intelligence" or HEI. This comes from the observation that humans build computers, humans' programs them and provides for the data (direct entry or through the IoT) and humans are the beneficiaries of the deliverable at all times (or should be).

I am re-branding "artificial intelligence" to "Human Enhanced Intelligence" or HEI

Giving the idea that HEI supercomputers can overcome the need of the human to program and enter data becoming independent agents, it should not hinder the possibility to harness the technology in a reasonable way with proper control systems. However, computers only have the information and logic processes provided by humans as well as learning routines, thus, they will not go too far in surpassing human intelligence in future developments.

Let me elaborate the concept of HEI or AI. Machines are not humans, nor living beings as we know it. Therefore, machines will not be able to have the human drive for survival and perpetuation. The sense of purpose is only going to be as good as the program itself that was envisioned by humans. That sense of purpose is influenced by factors that are not possible to rationalize and convert into a program that a computer can utilize effectively. I mean, humans are driven. We wake up every morning, go to work to provide for our loved ones, sometimes doing things that does not fulfill us professionally and seem not logical, but we do it because we are human.

Human sense of purpose is feed by the human drive that comes from many factors: survival, perpetuation, love, hate, empathy, sympathy, pain, passion, apathy, disdain, belief, bonds, societal perception, desire, self-satisfaction, etc, as well as the sense of mortality.

We cannot program a computer to love, because love is mostly illogical, since it involves selflessness, sacrifice and altruism. When a computer is programmed to perform a finite task, that task cannot be explained mathematically inferring sacrifice, or altruism as variables. Those will not allow the "procurement of the most successful outcome", and therefore could be construed as not-intelligent, or dumb.

Human intelligence is multifaceted, and only one aspect is computational (logic, mathematics, statistics, and data gathering and processing). Human intelligence also includes emotions and drives together with physiological and psychological needs and the senses. Out data inputs are more than what we read, see or hear. Our senses are not limited to the five recognized ones, therefore our data input for a task may have more variables than we consider as such for HEI.

The way humans rationalize concepts and arrive to conclusions are not only based on statistical approaches or algorithms, and the data we utilize is not only the one that we can convert into values for analysis. We sometimes use also gut feelings, take chances without reliable data, believe, follow orders without challenging, respect and obey.

The big difference between natural intelligence and "artificial intelligence" is that the latter one has access to discrete definable information instantaneously and the speed of analysis can be increased up to the point limit of the ability of the microprocessors to process. However, the data, the process and the hardware are human designed or defined and therefore an enhancement of the computational aspect of human intelligence.

Since the topic is very complex to elaborate in a simple article, and I am not an expert but an observer, let me focus on how AI or EHI can assist deliver excellent and timely HealthCare.

The data, the process and the hardware are human designed or defined and therefore an enhancement of the computational aspect of human intelligence.

Part II – EHI (AI) and HealthCare

Medical devices comprise less than 20% of the health care market, and diagnostic devices are at the forefront. Since computational power and data storage were very limited until recently, the medical device industry did not grow au par with the biopharmaceutical one. But things have changed. Medical devices are gaining momentum providing diagnostic power that was not seen ever. The ability to have a device "read" biopsy slides and compare them with thousands if not hundreds of thousands of qualified samples, will allow fast and accurate diagnosis and decision in human health. That is not only thanks to the ability of computers to store huge amounts of data, and the great processing power that allows fast rendering, but also to the crowdsourcing of ideas and concepts as well as data share that allows fast growth in the market. "Artificial intelligence" enhances doctor's capabilities to make decisions without the need of second test or analysis, reducing time to do consultations or research, since they are all embedded already into the systems.

Electronic health records (EHR) will also be a necessary step in the medicine of the future in which data share will allow more efficient delivery of care. Privacy protections will have to be enhanced to convince patients of the benefits.

In the very near future, we will be able to wear sensors (may be embedded in our garments) that communicate data directly to our EHR and proactive prevention of e.g. heart attacks, seizures, or obesity can be achieved. We can actually keep a tab on all possible known variables that may influence our state of health and have doctors proactively prevent disease.

Having the ability to deal with extensive health data, will provide better detection of disease signals that are not possible now unless we run a controlled clinical trial. The approach to medical research will change dramatically since subject enrolment will be procured instead of expected due to the ability to find potential participants or data momentarily.

The question is, will AI replace doctors? And my answer is, NO. Because the source of the knowledge always resides on humans, and the drive for better health care is to provide relief from pain and suffering as well as compassion that may not be interpreted by machines or understood mathematically.

The main goals of AI in health care should be the delivery of the best care possible to provide the most successful outcome. The final decision makers will always be the doctor and the patient, and that cannot be changed since it will impact human autonomy.

In conclusion, with the advent of this technology, humans should have full control on HEI or AI, at all times, providing for appropriate data and process algorithms in which axiomatic approach to the protection of human integrity, life and autonomy is provided. Constant controls should be embedded into the HEI or AI systems to detect and correct any deviations from the core principles for human protection. The differentiation between human and machine should be part of the system itself, where continuous tests (e.g. Turing test) are run to allow human control on the machine learning process and application of new knowledge. And the most important part is, that we should keep the mechanical power-off button accessible at all times, just in case...

Originally published on February 14, 2018

Clinical Trials Success Marred with 90% of Disappointment

It's been long said that the clinical trial process is costly and cumbersome and that regulatory requirements are too stringent to permit success in bringing a therapeutic product to the market. On the other hand, who would invest in an enterprise that has evidently demonstrated to fail in more than 90% of the cases? Well, large pharma companies as well as thousands of small start-ups are not deterred by the success rate. The rewards on having only one product reach the market, encourages risky investments that in the long term may yield great benefit.

The truth of the matter is that the process to determine the probability of success (POS) is contingent to access to accurate data and risk analysis. Accuracy of the data available to determine risk and POS lays on the knowledge base accrued during preclinical development, as well as having a robust knowledge of the disease and the intricate molecular basis of the disease in question. Further, an in-depth risk assessment will only provide an estimation of success based on previous experiences, and do not contemplate unknown risks that at the end are the most likely reason of failure.

Presently, risk assessments are embedded in the clinical trial process in a manner never seen before, where the new ICG GCP revision 2 prompts sponsors in assessing risk and managing risk during the entire process in a very well documented manner. Needless to say that risk assessments together with stringent requirements for quality assurance will only increase uncertainty.

But where I am heading to?

I want to rationalize why the success rates are so low in comparison with the investment and accrued knowledge to date. A paper published by A. W. Low et al. (2018) makes reason of success rates in drug development.

According to that paper, the overall POS from phase 1 to approval (1-APP) of the 15,102 drugs analyzed between years 2000-2016, phase to phase, is 6.9% for all indications analyzed, while for phase 3 to approval is 59%. Oncology drugs fare the worst with an overall POS of 3.4% (SE,0.2), while cardiovascular and vaccines fare the best with around 25% POS. Also, they demonstrated that the inclusion of biomarkers in clinical trials, increased the POS by almost 50% overall. When they analysed orphan drug development, they observed a similar tendency in POS. The authors also demonstrated that the POS did not change dramatically from year to year for the periods and diseases studied (actually, there was a decrease in the periods between 2007-2010 mostly due in my opinion, to the global economic downfall). However, they observed an increase of POS by almost half, for phase 3 studies in the period of 2014-2015, but with little overall impact.

> *"the overall POS from phase 1 to approval (1-APP) of the 15,102 drugs analyzed between years 2000-2016, phase to phase, is 6.9% for all indications"*

This paper definitively demonstrates that the POS of clinical trials is low compared to other business endeavours, and that overall, we are well below 10% success overall in a phase 1 to APP analysis up to 2015.

The reasons are very varied, and the data only depicts a reality that we are very well aware of, that the drug development process is very volatile, and that some improvements have been observed, but mainly in including study subjects that are considered, due to the use of biomarkers, to be the best candidates to favourably respond to treatment. Of course, that may not extrapolate to changes in prescription habits since the use of biomarkers is very limited.

"the inclusion of biomarkers in clinical trials, increased the POS by almost 50% overall"

It is very important to understand that the drug development process is extremely complex, since it is based on fundamental challenges of human nature, and that new candidates are only identified in function of marketability and revenues (ROI).

"more resources and investments are not translated into new drugs"

It is time to implement a new paradigm in clinical research, where candidates are identified and pursue through development based on the very principles of beneficence, ethics and patient safety. Also, it is important to understand that more resources and investments are not translated into new drugs (i.e. oncology drug development), and that depending on the point of view of success, we may not really have great drugs, but just good enough.

Originally published on March 16, 2018

Bringing the hospital care home, a feasible solution for tackling health care costs and promote better outcomes

I was just recently reviewing some data regarding the projections of health care costs in the near future due to the fact that our population is aging and that baby boomers are retiring. There is a considerable interest on forecasting the possible liabilities and reduce expenditures, since population growth in the western hemisphere is stagnated and the pyramid of population looks more like upside down, having fewer younger people footing the bill of a large number of older peers.

The common notion that health are costs are going to increase is based on the fact that analysts are just extrapolating costs in function of the classic systems for delivering care. In Canada for example, health care costs increased a whooping 70% in the last two decades, while delivery of care has not. In the US, for example, health care costs increased three-fold since 1960, or an 18.2% of the GDP. In this case we have to consider that in the US about 50% of care is delivered privately, what may compound the cost even further. The average cost per capita of health care in the US is double than most of the developed countries (together with Switzerland).

We cannot expect to have a solution without looking outside of the box. Delivery of care as it is now, is not sustainable and something has to be done.

One very plausible solution is to streamline critical and acute care to hospitals, and chronic care outside of hospitals. One study (1) was done a long time ago to compare outcomes of hospital at home care versus hospital care, and observed no differences generally, moreover, patients were happier to recover at home. Also, the Cochrane Database of Systematic Reviews, Hospital at home versus in-patient hospital care (2), observed that patients admitted to hospital at home did not generally have significantly different outcomes than those treated in hospital. This study questions the healthcare savings from the point of view of the patients in focus, however, does not estimate the release of hospital beds to other acute patients who might need care. However, just this August, a study (3a) concluded that hospital home care delivery as 30-day episode of post acute transitional care, generally improved outcomes measured in function of acute period length of stay, all-cause 30-day hospital readmission and ED visits, admissions to skilled nursing facilities (SNFs), referral to a certified home health care agency, and patient experiences with care.

The reality is that we cannot increase the number of hospital beds to infinity, as we cannot have an unlimited budget to face future care needs, and also, we cannot provide high quality care in an environment of financial constraint where staff overworked, and burnout is the norm.

Therefore, the solution is very simple. First is prevention to reduce the number of patients that require care.

Let's look at diabetes. According to the American Diabetes Association, in 2015, 30.3 million Americans, or 9.4% of the population, had diabetes. Of the 30.3 million adults with diabetes,

23.1 million were diagnosed, and 7.2 million were not diagnosed. Diabetes remains the 7th leading cause of death in the United States in 2015. Total costs of diagnosed diabetes in the United States in 2017 was $327 billion. Further, the economic costs of diabetes increased by 26% from 2012 to 2017 due to the increased prevalence of diabetes and the increased cost per person with diabetes. When health care costs were analyzed per disease, (3), type -2 diabetes is leading with a total of $101.4 billion dollars in 2013. Global prevalence of the disease is estimated to increase from 2.8 in the year 2000 to 4.4% in 2030 (4). The most important data is also that there is an increase of patients in the age group 65 years and older that are being diagnosed with diabetes.

Type 2 diabetes is preventable and possibly reversible with lifestyle changes that include exercise, reduction of body weight and smoking cessation. Treatment and follow up of diabetic patients in their homes will not only improve the outcomes but reduce an overall financial burden to the society at large.

To implement a system that supports Hospital at Home Care we should first establish:

- a policy to allow health care systems streamline patients with chronic conditions to hospital at home
- create a medical sub specialty for hospital at home care where areas as oncology, geriatrics, neonatology, psychiatry, social medicine are further enhanced
- create a nursing sub specialty that addresses as above
- create a professional home health care specialist with knowledge and experience to assist patients at home
- provide for a streamlined approach to triage to hospital at home care, with seamless transition and minimum patient inconvenience, regardless whether they were previously hospitalized or not.

This type of approach is already being implemented with good results (5). Allowing patients to be treated at home (when possible) will certainly reduce infrastructure costs and promote better outcomes.

The availability of wearable medical devices with full connectivity through smartphone applications will allow doctors and nurses follow up on their patients on real time and prompt care when needed.

In 2016 U.S. health care spending increased 4.3 percent to reach $3.3 trillion, or $10,348 per person (6). Hospital care amounts for 34% of the expenditure. In Canada, on the other hand in 2017 the total health care expenditure was $ 242 billion, or $ 6,604 per person. Hospital care amounted for 28.3% of the total health care budget (7). Hospital costs are estimated to grow between 2-4% annually. Promoting hospital at home care, may provide of great impact to the health care budgets, and improve outcomes.

Originally published on October 16, 2018

(1) BMJ. 1998 Jun 13; 316(7147): 1786–1791.

(2) https://www.cochranelibrary.com/cdsr/doi/10.1002/14651858.CD000356.pub2/abstract

(3) JAMA. 2016;316(24):2627-2646. doi:10.1001/jama.2016.16885

(3a) JAMA Intern Med. 2018;178(8):1033-1040. doi:10.1001/jamainternmed.2018.256

(4) https://doi.org/10.2337/diacare.27.5.1047

(5) https://www.stjoes.ca/our-stories/news/~1860-Integrated-Comprehensive-Care-reduces-hospital-length-of-stay-costs-for-patients-with-chronic-diseases

(6) https://www.cms.gov/Research-Statistics-Data-and-Systems/Statistics-Trends-and-Reports/NationalHealthExpendData/downloads/highlights.pdf

(7) https://www.cihi.ca/sites/default/files/document/nhex2017-trends-report-en.pdf

Quality Management and Risk in Clinical Trials - New GCP R2 Revision

Good Clinical Practices (ICH – GCP) is the cornerstone in the standardization of the clinical research process since its implementation in 1995. Identifying the three main players on the clinical research process (ethics committees, sponsors and investigators), allowed the construct of an entire scaffolding in which the parties could build processes and procedures to ensure that all controls and protections are considered. Of course, the guideline was originally written in 1990's, where all the processes were paper based, and mostly studies were run in one country or region. Things have changed since then, and Information Technology is taking the lead in the clinical research process.

GCP did not come without challenges, being the first one, in my opinion, the qualification and function of ethics committees (EC). GCP established roles and responsibilities of EC, however, a long time had to pass until some understanding of their key role was achieved. Principal investigators are the second party involved in clinical trials for which GCP has precise responsibilities. Conversely, the major changes in the guideline of 2016 came for the clinical trial sponsors QA process.

Clinical Trial Sponsors are now responsible to implement a Quality Management System that is intrinsically proportionate to the risk of the study and the importance of the data collected.

In the original version of GCP, it was already established that a risk assessment is part of the quality system for clinical trial conduct. However, it was left up to the interpretation of the sponsor and their ability to meet their responsibilities effectively.

While teaching Clinical Development for the last 20 years, I included risk assessment as a key learning part in the process of determining project management approaches to clinical trials. Risk assessment was already inherent to the project management process even before the revision. However, implementation was very limited, since it adds cost to the clinical research enterprise. On the other hand, we can observe that there are well established quality management processes for medical devices, for instance, that may very easily be applied to drug development to avoid the reinvention of the wheel. Nonetheless, that will add much more cost to the development of new drugs.

Focusing on the aspect of Risk Management in clinical research, we should look into what GCP R2 establishes. The risk-based approach was primarily introduced to allow central monitoring gain a position of acceptability in the practice of clinical trials management, and therefore all the new risk assessment strategies formulated are a validation of already implemented processes taking place.

The establishment of Risk Management in within the sponsors QMS as per GCP includes seven individually defined processes as follows:

1. Identification of critical processes and data to ensure subject protection and data reliability (5.0.1)

2. Risk identification (systemic and trial based) (5.0.2)

3. Risk Evaluation (new risks against established controls) (5.0.3)

4. Risk Control (mitigation and acceptability of risks) (5.0.4)

5. Risk Communication (provision of risk management documentation to allow continuous review and assessment of risk) (5.0.5)

6. Risk Review (periodic review and update) (5.0.6)

7. Risk Reporting (description of QMS and deviations in CSR) (5.0.7)

Risk assessment was also introduced at the level of data management and systems validation (5.5.3). At that level, the data management professionals should look into the new ISO 13485:2016 in which controls and risk assessment processes for medical device and associated software development is very well established.

Evidently, the risk management requirements in clinical trials add a new level of complexity in defining the risks and establishing controls for clinical trials and QMS that need critical expertise. That expertise is not readily available in the clinical development arena, since it was not critical in the past. Then, the focus was put mainly on hands-on monitoring as established in the past version of GCP, and QA to determine adherence to protocol and standard operational procedures.

Readiness to comply with this new requirement will determine which sponsors will be able to progress and make use of the new processes effectively in order to determine good drug candidates early in development.

The cost of implementing the new ICG GCP E2 was not clearly estimated yet. In my opinion, it will impact development greatly leaving the playing field only to the ones who are ready.

Our company is ready to assist familiarize your professionals on these changes that impact profoundly on how clinical trials business is done. Just contact me for more information.

Originally published on January 17, 2018

Registry Studies and RWD taking the lead in Clinical Research

For the last three decades, double blind randomized placebo controlled trials (RCT) were the "gold standard" for pharmaceutical research. Anything that did not fit the standard was considered "unreliable data", and therefore subject to heavy scrutiny. The reality of the matter is, that RCT data is a depiction of an ideal scenario of drug response in function of exceptionally staged conditions very far from what the real clinical setting is. That staging provoked an overwhelming increase in the cost of doing research due to the huge number of controls and assurance steps to maintain the study within constraints of its own virtuality. As a result, in some cases, we could not replicate the observed response in the real world, rendering the safety and effectiveness of certain product just virtual.

Observational research and registries intend to bring some reality to RCT as to understand drug response in the real clinical setting of a patient in their own environment with little or no controls. In some cases, observational studies were able to bring light to the most efficient intervention for a particular condition that affects millions of patients worldwide and, on the other hand, demystify certain interventions as not better than no treatment at all.

Efficiency of treatment interventions is not measured only with clinical variables of drug response, but also include other variables as important as the clinical ones as for instance, how easy it is for the patient to comply, or how fast the patient can return to normal activities, and how costly access to treatment is, to mention some.

Registries should take a front seat in clinical development since they shed real light into the efficiency of treatment interventions, in which patient centricity plays a key role. In my opinion, the patient should be the main source of data to determine if a treatment intervention is worth the cost and effort.

Our professional opinions are not significant in determining efficiency of a treatment intervention, if patients continue to be limited in their ability to return to certain normality, or their own opinion does not concur with ours.

Information technology applications and mHealth has brought to us an unprecedented number of tools to start collecting RWD (Real Wold Data). Data processing power is now suitable, allowing us render results fast. Social media platforms may help reduce the cost to implement data collection, and real time analysis would provide health care providers with a periodical update on the efficiency of treatment interventions. Further, artificial intelligence may allow us find more efficient avenues to determine optimal treatment interventions.

Registries and RWD should join the "gold standard" place to determine efficiency of treatment interventions, in which patient centricity plays a key role in the design of data collection protocols. Furthermore, pharmaco-economics and HEOR should join the clinical research position they deserve to provide more accurate visions on exceptional treatment interventions.

It would be great to hear your opinions on the issue, since all parties should join the conversation in defining a new paradigm of pharmaceutical product development.

Originally published on January 15, 2018

The dawn of The Body of all Knowledge, The natural evolution of Big Data

Everyone that is involved in science and analytics has been impacted by the new concept of big data. The notion seems to be that with the ability to collect and store never before possible amounts of data into data systems and further analyze it, would bring humanity to the next evolutionary step. However, the concept of big data as presented by the majority of its enthusiasts is far from being the next library of Alexandria created by Ptolemy I and dedicated to the Muses.

The ability to collect, store, and further analyze massive amounts of data should allow us to understand about human activity better (business, health, entertainment, science, etc.). We might be able to forecast outcomes more precisely to avoid catastrophes and other misfortunes. The impression is that big data would allow us avoid big mistakes, making informed decisions about our future, understand the past and improve the present. However, the concept of big data is created on feeble assumptions.

First, I could not stop worrying that over 90% of all the data in the world was created in the last 2 years. Two years in humanity just reflects a spec of what we know or are able to perceive. That represent all values, texts, words, images, movies, etc. Especially this last two years there was no major discoveries or human advances in science and medicine, no major breakthroughs but were marred with crises and conflicts. But in 2 years we were able to fill 90% of the existing databases and is growing. It is perplexing that, thanks to mobile technology and user data driven systems, every day we create as much information as done since the beginning of time to 2003, that the amount of data created and stored by the industry doubles every 1.2 years, that Google alone processes on average over 40 thousand search queries per second, making it over 3.5 billion in a single day, that every minute we send more than 200 million emails, generate 1,8 million Facebook likes, send 278 thousand Tweets, and up-load 200 thousand photos to Facebook, in which around 100 hours of video are uploaded to YouTube every minute that would take one person about 15 years to watch every video uploaded by users in one single day, also that Facebook users share 30 billion pieces of content between them every day, and 570 new websites spring into existence every minute of every day. Of course, that is a fraction of big data, being automatic sensory systems and images the leading source. Basically, big data has the intention to include every bit of information captured from any source, stored in large data silos with the potential of being analyzed and further utilized for the seeming betterment of humanity.

It is prudent to stop at this point and make very exhaustive clarification of the main feebleness of big data. The weak links are the source of the data, reliability of the source and the analytics tools that are purpose driven.

In this article, as a response to many enthusiastic articles, I am discussing the source of data as presented in big data as complex and very heterogeneous. Data sources generally collects images, text and values and others content, all that is either user driven or electronically captured by "sensor" systems.

The big data concept is challenged by the data itself and how it is captured, handled, stored and further processed. The main issue about data is QUALIFICATION.

DATA QUALIFICATION

Data to be utilized in analysis as the basis of decision-making process must be previously QUALIFIED. Data qualification means that the source has to be determined as truthful and the veracity has to be documented further than a declaration from the data entry person, before the information is used to make sound decisions. Qualification may imply giving data different levels of veracity and therefore utilize it at your own risk. For example, Facebook likes are just perceptions that a virtual end user may have about something that was presented on her/his page on a given time point. As a perception is inherently biased, therefore of relative value. The end user may also be a 5 years old kid playing with the parent's computer and answering to a survey at random.

Qualification should also imply the elimination of:

REITERATION. Reiteration has to be eliminated before analysis. For example, one single picture can be tweeted, retweeted, re-retweeted, generate newspaper articles, discussions forums, blogs, arguments, images, movies, YouTube videos, etc. generating terabytes of information regardless of the relevance, all that from that one picture. It seems that there is a lot of data regarding a particular item or event, but is nothing more than the same thing repeated again and again. Utilization of repeated information that has originally only one or few sources is of weak evidence value yet can be artificially qualified as worthy of analysis. (Beware, "a lie repeated many times may become an accepted truth, nevertheless is a lie").

MISREPRESENTATION. Data collected for a particular purpose should not be repurposed since it might become a misrepresentation of the original data source. I will present a very rudimentary example to define misrepresentation: a company collects data regarding smells and which is the most liked. The majority of the people, having been given several options, choose chocolate cookie smell. If that data is used by a perfume company as guiding principle for a new product, they may consider that the analytics driven decision is to manufacture a new perfume that smells like cookies. The issue here was that the purpose of the data collection was to determine which smell people like the most when they enter a house that does not translate definitively to what people loves to smell in a perfume.

FALSE DATA. Data purposely created false. We can take as an example a novel or a sci-fi book about time travel that is stored in big data in a very redundant manner. Although my example is naïve, it could be interpreted as that either time travel is possible and/or the morlocks actually exist living in caves underground. Making a mining company who used the wrong data set regarding security risks invest in security and warfare to combat morlocks.

BIAS. Data can be entered in systems purposely created to guide the user to a particular conclusion to further benefit some groups, or intentionally damaging others. It is very important that the architecture created for data storage does not inherently bias the user towards a particular conclusion. For instance, let's assume that for an analysis of personal income only male earners data has been entered from the 1900s to the 1960s. This data will be biased based on gender, because in that period of time the majority of earners were male and limited or unreliable data exists for females, which can yield wrong conclusions on the general evolution of income.

TRANSFORMATION. Data could be transformed in the storage systems when transfer and backups are made, for which random unintentional transformations may yield to a silo of bad data. Big data systems must be qualified as the data itself. Reliability of the information as well as the containers have to be qualified before data analysis and further use to make decisions.

SELF-GENERATION. When data is processed, generates more data, which in turn will be reprocessed to generate more data, and so on and so forth. The use of data that is not from an original source (human or digital) but as a result of previous analytics, can be very unreliable since the ability to draw conclusion is based on premises and hypothesis that can be true or false. Utilizing data that was created using false hypotheses may draw us to further wrong conclusions that will be amplified exponentially every time a derivative from the original data is used.

RELEVANCE. Images or posts or tweets in a nonsensical manner. Data for the sake of data is not what all this is about. We can fill books with pages written with gibberish, and still pretend to have data silos that could be analyzed. Data relevance has to be established before considered qualified.

POOLING. Pooling data for further analysis when the original does not yield an answer as sought can inherently enter bias and errors. Statistically there are accepted approaches to data pooling, however in big data, we might have to redefine pooling approaches to avoid deviations from the truth.

SECURITY. Data has to be secure to avoid hacking.

STABILITY. Data has to be accessible at all times and the flow of data cannot be hindered by lack of capabilities of infrastructures created in lieu of big data

LEGACY. Data access has to be guaranteed in time to avoid losing information due to changes in system architecture, language, configurations and updates.

READABILITY. All data has to be readable with universal readers therefore big data has to be stored in a universal storage format that can be built upon in the future.

ACCESS. All people should have the privilege to access publicly generated big data as an evidence of transparency. Like having a library card, we can enter the library and read as far as are in good standing.

In conclusion, the concept of big data is a very limited one as to representing the capabilities of humanity in developing or seeing beyond the scope of our senses in function of technological capabilities developed in the last decade. Intuition will be replaced and/or enhanced by relevant hard evidence. Big data should be interpreted as raw, and is not the solution itself to a better understanding of information for the purpose aforesaid.

Large amounts of data have to be properly qualified and relevant, free from reiterations, misrepresentations, false data, transformations and bias, cannot be self-generating, or result of pooling of unreliable elements. Also data has to be secure from malicious attacks at all times, the systems must be stable and audit trails should be generated and preserved for future search. Readability and access should be also guaranteed at all times. Once data and data systems pass through all the rigours of a qualification process, it can be used for purpose driven analytics or mining, torturing or whatever the user considers necessary to identify new trends, or forecast possible events. Properly qualified data will then be part of the Body of all Knowledge (phonetically: BooK) that will grow truthfully in time.

Therefore, the concept of big data should be replaced by Body of all Knowledge, on which the users will be assured of the reliability of information and knowledge generated with such information. As it stands now, is just a lot of clutter.

Originally published on February 25, 2015. LinkedIn as an Opinion Paper

Index

Adaptive design, 126, 129
ADR, 53
Adverse Event Reporting, 53
AE, 53, 54, 55, 56, 57, 58
Artificial Intelligence, 175
Catch 22, 31
catch-22, 20, 21, 24
Centrally based, 127
Clinical research, 11, 12, 31, 158
Clinical Research, 15, 21, 22, 25, 28, 31, 37, 49, 50, 69, 83, 87, 95, 97, 117, 135, 137, 141, 143, 145, 193
Clinical Trials Monitor, 43
Comparable Experience, 34
COMPARABLE EXPERIENCE, 35
Compliance Monitoring and Data verification, 60
Consenting Clinical Trial Subjects, 169
CRA, 21, 22, 34, 59, 60, 93, 126, 127, 128, 129, 130, 135, 143, 144
CROs, 21, 28, 94, 135
declaration of Helsinki, 16, 122
Depression, 149
Direct Experience, 34
DIRECT EXPERIENCE, 35
Drug dispensing, 73
drug safety, 3, 39, 40, 41, 42

EFFECTIVE MARKETING, 42
Efficacy endpoints, 113
Efficacy vs. Efficiency, 99
EFFICIENCY, 102, 103
ePRO, 69, 70, 71, 72, 74, 134, 147
Ethical monitoring, 60
GCP, 11, 20, 22, 23, 33, 35, 54, 60, 72, 93, 94, 98, 135, 141, 167, 168, 182, 189, 190, 191, 192
Good Clinical Practices, 11, 16, 53, 59, 117, 118, 122, 138, 140, 167
Health Care Crisis, 159
healthy volunteer, 121, 123
Home based, 127
hospital care, 185, 186
In house based, 127
Investigational Drugs, 111
Job Interview, 77, 91
Medical Monitoring, 59, 60
monitoring the clinical trial, 59
Nursing, 141
Opioid overdose, 165
Patient Centered Care, 146
Patient Centered Medicine, 145, 146
Patient Centric Medicine, 145, 147
PATIENT EDUCATION, 41

PATIENT UNIQUENESS, 41
perception of risk, 39, 42
Personalized Medicine, 145, 147
pharmaceutical companies, 15, 21, 28, 171
Placebo Effect, 105
Pregnancy, 151, 157
Project Manager, 49, 50
Quality Management, 189, 190
Registry Studies, 193
Relevant Experience, 32
RELEVANT EXPERIENCE, 35
Remote based, 127
RISK, 40
Risk in Clinical Trials, 189
RWD, 193, 194

Safety Monitoring, 60, 61
Social media, 71, 194
Subject consenting, 74
Subject enrollment, 72
Subject randomization, 73
Subject selection, 71
Subject visits., 74
The Clinical Research Associate or Monitor, 21
The Clinical Research Coordinator, 22, 143
The Clinical Research Scientist, 22
The Monitor, 21, 60
Training, 22, 87, 142
Virtually based, 127
volunteer positions, 29
Volunteering vs. entry level job, 30
Volunteering vs. Internship, 29

www.ingramcontent.com/pod-product-compliance
Lightning Source LLC
Chambersburg PA
CBHW051308220526
45468CB00004B/1261